Health-Warrior

Fighting for your health and well-being

Dr DJEMAL U. SINDELI

First Edition

Copyright © 2007 Djemal U. Sindeli

The moral right of the author has been asserted.

All rights reserved. No part of this publication may be produced, stored in a retrival system, or transmitted, in any form or by any means, without prior permission in writing of the publisher, nor be otherwise circulated in any form of binding or cover other than that which it is published and without a similar condition including this condition being imposed on the subsequent purchaser.

ISBN 978 1 84799 767 8

Health-Warrior website: health-warrior.co.uk
Email: info@health-warrior.co.uk

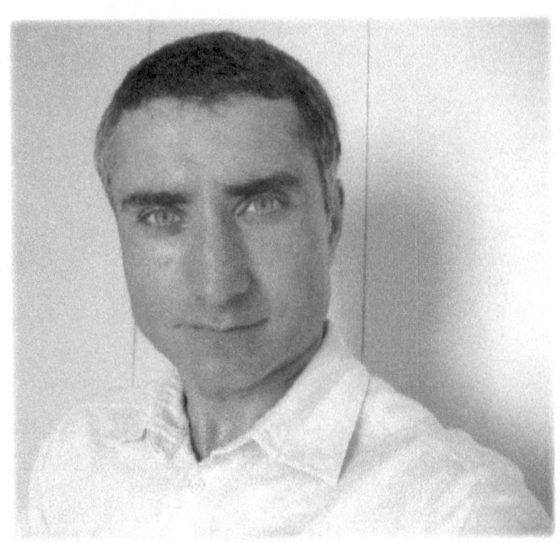

About the author

Djemal is an internationally renowned and successful wellness consultant, personal trainer, and health and fitness scholar. After successfully completing his doctorate, covering human health and nutrition, and specialising in physical activity, he went on to establish two consulting companies: Motion Fitness and Sena wellness.

Djemal is dedicated to bringing public attention to the link between health and lifestyle propaganda and human illness and disease. He is recognized as a wellness activist, viewed as a health and fitness contrarian, and a physical activity guru.

Health-Warrior was born after the culmination of more than two decades of consulting, training, and coaching. Its mission is to empower, inspire, and motivate and take you on the road to a better health and well-being.

He resides with his wife and family in a traditional town home, which sits on lofty location overlooking the Mediterranean coast.

Contact details: djemal@health-warrior.co.uk

Author's note

Health-Warrior is intended solely for educational and information purposes, and not as medical advice.

Human vulnerability to disease cannot be reduced to one single physical or psychological cause. Many genetic, nutritional, environmental, emotional and other known factors contribute to illness and disease.

Neither the publishers nor the author can accept responsibility for injuries or illness arising out of a failure by the reader to consult a qualified medical or health professional with any questions concerning their health.

Contents

Introduction

The fight back for your optimum health and well-being starts here. The Health-Warrior will give you the knowledge and practical solutions, to transform your life. You will reclaim and rejuvenate what is rightfully yours: a healthy mind and body. The emphasis is on optimizing your health and wellness today to prevent the health problems of tomorrow.

> **Health-Warrior/** hel`th-wa`ri`or / noun [C] /
> a person who tries to stop damage to human health and well-being

Too often, people are 'too busy' to address the health and well-being concerns of themselves or their family. The nature of modern living means that a person will attract higher stress levels, be less likely to be physically active, and more likely to make unhealthy nutritional and lifestyle choices. The impacts and consequences of not investing the appropriate time and effort into optimising personal physical and emotional wellness, can weigh heavily on your daily life and the lives of your loved ones. Any loss in quality of life because of emotional and physical damage will eventually open the door to injury, illness, or disease.

Good health is the most important thing in life, even if it is not always seen as important as, money for example. It is the case however; that in the event of a person suffering a debilitating injury, illness, or disease, they would willingly return the money they have accumulated in their life, just to secure the return of their good health. Unfortunately, in most cases, this is not an option, and not all the money in the world would reunite them with their good health, once it has failed.

The Health-Warrior will assist and provide for you the unique opportunity to focus on transformational life changes, changes that will improve your physical, mental, and emotional health. Proactive solutions gleaned from the Health-Warrior will ensure high levels of health; increases in emotional and physical energy, escalating vitality, creativity, and youthful living.

Nature imitates herself. A grain thrown into good ground brings forth fruit; a principle thrown into a good mind brings forth fruit. Everything is created and conducted by the same Master, the root, the branch, the fruits: the principles, the consequences.

Pascal

Fighting for your health and well-being
Do you have a choice to lead a life of full of optimum health, happiness, and fulfilment? If you live in a politically stable democratic country with sound environmental, socioeconomic foundations, earn a regular income, and enjoy your liberty then you might be forgiven for thinking (and even arguing) that the choice is yours. In fact, your health nurturing choices are being limited to the ones other people would like you to follow. You are guided down a path that is as profitable for some, as it is detrimental to others, and you.

The Health-Warrior, in taking you on a journey to a life of optimum health, happiness, and fulfilment, will also seek to explode the 'choice is yours' myth by introducing you to the forces actively trying to move you away from optimum health, moreover, making it a daily fight just to maintain the health you have.

In view of the extensive reach of these forces, to try to live a healthy and happy life in today's world, necessitates an enormous amount of self-control and considerable discipline; those who are influenced and only able to offer a minimal resistance to these forces of ill health, are on the road to self-destruction. The Health-Warrior was born to stand up against these forces, and by doing so empower you to stop any further damage to your health, and promote new ways of living to maximise it.

The goal of every person should be to attain a maximum quality of life; one that reduces the risks of premature aging of body cells, is illness-free, and supports the body functions that give physical and psychological vitality, energy, and zest.

Health-Warrior

During the many years I consulted, and continue to consult and coach clients, on their health and well-being, it is clear to me that people searching for a better quality of life, firstly need to be aware that there is an ongoing battle to secure it. Secondly, they need to know, who it is they are fighting against, and finally, they need to have a proven strategy to fight back against them. The battle for a healthy life is so heavily stacked against a person, that instead of continually striving and achieving a better quality of life, their conscious, or unconscious poor choices take them down dark alleys of temporary or permanent illness and disease.

Seeking solutions
The one outstanding thought I carry around with me while talking to anyone about health and well-being, is the fact that the body is a beautifully balanced creation, full of immeasurable wonders that operate with a fascinating simplicity and admirable complexity. It is obvious to me that the body, or its functions, cannot ever be isolated or viewed as parts and sections; it can only be viewed as a whole.

It is at its most basic, a humble atom, and a plentiful assortment of chemical reactions. The body seeks a balanced state; the physicist, Sir Isaac Newton explained, 'for every action there is an equal and opposite reaction'. The body is no exception to this rule, with every one of your actions, be it the consumption of air, water, food or chemical supplements, your body will supply a suitable equal and opposite reaction; and do its best to maintain the perfect operating equilibrium. Complex physiological systems determine the conditions under which you exhibit human need such as the need for food or water. This process is referred to as homeostasis; derived from the Latin words 'homeo' meaning same or similar and 'stasis' meaning 'equilibrium or balance'; it is an internal mechanism by which the body maintains internal biological systems under variable environmental stresses. Among the important homeostatic systems of the body are the ones that regulate blood pressure, blood cell production, blood sugar, and metabolism.

In each part of the Health-Warrior, you will discover how your choices to live a life full of optimum health, happiness, and fulfilment are being eroded and diminished. Moreover, you will discover how to fight back to reclaim the perfect balance for your physical, emotional, and optimum health and well-being.

Further information about the Health-Warrior can be viewed at website:
health-warrior.co.uk

Part one

Air power

Oxygen is critical in maintaining a superior quality of life, as it affects all your activities. Your thoughts, feelings, and actions come from the energy generated by it, accounting for approximately 90% of your total energy. Furthermore, 60% of your body is composed of it. It is, without exaggeration, the most essential and vital element of your life.

In both developed and rapidly industrialising countries, the major historic air pollution problem has typically been high levels of smoke and sulphur dioxide, arising from the combustion of sulphur-containing fossil fuels such as coal for domestic and industrial purposes. The major threat to clean air is now posed by traffic emissions. Petrol and diesel engine motor vehicles emit a wide variety of pollutants, which have an increasing impact on urban air quality. In addition, further reactions with sunlight on these vehicle pollutants leads to the formation of ozone, a secondary long-range pollutant, which affects many areas often far from the original emission site. Acid rain is another long-range pollutant influenced by vehicle emissions. With pollution from traffic sources continuing to increase and the world population expanding unabated, there is a growing need for more and more energy. Consequently, greater levels of pollution are leaving behind worsening levels of air quality, with less clean air to be distributed among an increasing number of people.

By reducing the 'pollution footprint' you leave on this Earth, optimising the quality of air you breathe, and refining the actual process of breathing, you will discover ways in which you can really make a difference in your life. Unleash a 'new' you, with transformations such as increased energy, vitality, and mental focus. With the additional benefits of reduced stress levels, strengthened immune system, renewed body parts, and invigorated body functions, and the subduing, and in some cases, the reversing of premature aging.

It is a life giving and sustaining element; give it the appropriate gratitude and above all, attention.

Chapter 1

Air Essentials

Oxygen was introduced to the world around two billion years ago, and the first plant life appeared soon after. Other forms of life found it hard to cope with the new toxic element. As many years passed, animal and human existence hinged on their ability to adapt to this oxygen challenge. Thankfully, evolutionary adaptations created an efficient way to use the oxygen for energy production.

Body basics
The energy production took place in the mitochondria (also known as calorie-burning machines) found in human cells. It proved so successful that oxygen has become the powerhouse behind most of the body processes that fuel life. Your life depends on your ability to breathe and provide the oxygen to these mitochondria. Oxygen is essential to all life; the quality of your breathing and your ability to utilise it will determine how energetic a life you will lead. Each breath creates, protects, and sustains your life, but how well it does so is determined by how efficient your respiratory system performs. Make simple lifestyle changes and you can improve your ability to make conscious healthful improvements to your body and mind, achieving measurable results and immeasurable natural bliss.

The average person will breathe around 12 breaths per minute and take in half a litre to a litre of air. The breathing function is controlled by interaction of the brainstem and the cortical in the spinal pathways. The brainstem looks after those occasions when automatic control is necessary, such as when you are sleeping or unconscious, and the cortical takes up responsibilities when you are awake.

Before reaching the lungs, you will purify, warm, and humidify the air you breathe in through your nose. Under normal breathing, the air is heated up to body temperature and its humidity increased by more than 90% in the nose area. This heated and humidified air is drawn into 2,300km of airways, followed by hundreds of millions of alveoli (where the oxygen in the air is deposited into your body in exchange for carbon dioxide).

The breathing cycle can be separated into four stages:

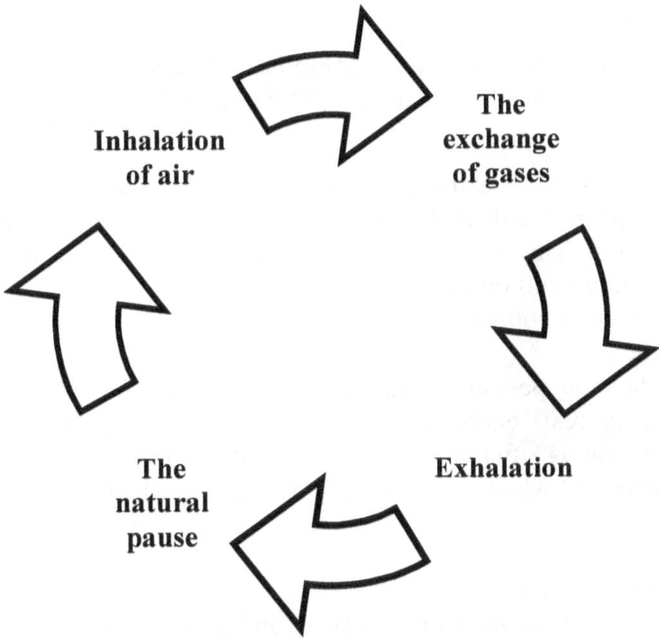

For respiration, the skeletal muscles are an essential component. The diaphragm can be compared to a piston of a car engine that is operating in the mid part of the chest. The rib cage acts as the cylinder that the piston pushes down into, and the piston is attached to the lungs by an elastic coil. As the piston pushes down, air is sucked into your lungs and the natural reflex of the elastic coil pulls (without the need for other muscles) the piston back, causing the outward breath.

When you cough, these respiratory muscles are called into action and can propel the air out at 10 litres per seconds, and even faster when you sneeze!

When a person performs physical activity however, the additional muscles, abdominal (stomach), and intercostals (in between the ribs) are recruited to help with breathing out. For a physically active person, moderate activity would elevate the breathing rate to 30 breaths per minute, 50 per minute if performing more vigorous activity; moreover, up to 100 breaths per minute when suffering from serious stress.

The average adult has a lung size of four to six litres, about the size of a basketball and weighs one kilogram; and most amazing of all, if taken from the body and spread out, it would cover over half a tennis court. All this, and you never exceed 60% of your vital capacity.

Every breath you take

> Everyone is trying to accomplish something big, not realizing that life is made up of little things.
>
> *Frank A. Clarke*

If you watch a child breathe while they sleep, you will notice that their abdomen is pushed out as they inhale and then sucked back in as they exhale. Their upper chest and ribcage are almost motionless. It is the perfect technique and one that adults should seek to replicate. It is ironic that the occasions you breathe best are the times when least aware of it, such as sleeping.

A healthy person should breathe in a manner that seems most natural during rest, exercise, and recovery. Breathing, being a most natural function is often incorrectly performed, taken for granted and totally overlooked when a person seeks to improve their health and well-being.

Wisdom from the past

The acts of breathing, its study, practice, and positive effects on physical and mental well-being go back thousands of years. The concept of life energy is a universal one, and evidence of shared knowledge regarding this philosophy on health can be found among all the ancient cultures. The sources stretch from east to west and north to south, but they all share similar discoveries and words of wisdom. These irreplaceable gifts have been handed down through hundreds of generations, and given that the physiology of the body has changed little in this time, it allows you to use these gifts to benefit your health and well-being.

> The human body may not have changed very much but the damaging effects of the environment on the human body have.
>
> *Health-Warrior*

The people of India past, viewed breathing as an art, to be practiced and perfected. The breath of life was a masterpiece, which was a perpetual work in progress. Their belief was that breath, life, and energy were fundamentally connected to each other, and gave all three the single word of 'prana'. Pranayama, where the breathing was proactively managed, saw increased vitality, mental abilities, and holistic awareness.

The breath acted as the link to the nervous system. The benefits could be accumulated through practice and development of breathing techniques; maximising a fantastic source of energy with simplicity being the ultimate advantage. They lived with the adage that 'the better you breathe, the better you feel' and they were ultimately seeking a 'natural bliss'.

The Bhagavad-Gita is an historical Indian poem, which is an introduction into the ancient culture of India, demonstrates these beliefs further. Thoughts and emotions were implicitly linked to breathing: 'draw in their breath to feed the flame of thought, and breathe it forth to waft the heart on high'. The following quotation has been viewed as the humans ability to self-heal and live a balanced and illness-free life: 'Offering inhaling breath into the outgoing breath, and offering the outgoing breath into the inhaling breath, the Yogi neutralises both these breaths; He thus releases the life force from the heart and brings it under his control'.

In the Autobiography of a Yogi, while in conversation with his mentor, the Yogi is told that 'A sweet new breath of divine hope will penetrate the arid hearts of worldly men' and is the 'Breath which binds the soul to the body'. The yogi, later in his journey of discovery, explains his thoughts on the importance of the body's need to rest and its subconscious abilities for renewal. 'Sleep is rejuvenating due to man's temporary unawareness of body and breath. The sleeping man becomes a Yogi. Unconsciously releasing him to the healing brain and spinal cord centres.'

> Your breathing is a reflection of your emotions; breathe happiness into your life and reduce the negative emotions of anger, frustration, anxiety, fear, worry, and panic.
>
> *Health-Warrior*

Some Indian Yogis believe you are given a set number of breaths at birth, and if you can learn to use your breath more efficiently, you will use less from your allotted life-quota, and therefore age at a slower pace and live longer. They use the tortoise as an example, as it breathes at four breaths per minute and can reach the age of 300!

> Breathing activities can be performed anywhere and at anytime, and gives you the power to live with increased energy, vitality, and mental focus; reduced stress levels; strengthened immune system; renewed body parts and invigorated functions; reversed premature aging.
>
> *Health-Warrior*

Ch'i is the Chinese word for 'life energy' and is the vibrancy that electrifies all living things; and the more you accumulate the healthier you will be. Your stream of physical, psychological, and emotional well-being flows freely and clear of blockages and stagnation. Your ch'i is managed by precise methods of breathing, mental focus and imagery.

Ch'i Kung is the further development of the life energy. Early practices and activities of Ch'i Kung, which translated means 'working with the energy of life', date as far back as 1028BC. It is a holistic approach, which encompasses posture, movement, self-massage, meditation, and breathing activities, with an undertaking to learn how to manage the flow and distribution of ch'i to improve the health and harmony of the mind and body. The Chinese applied Ch'i Kung to prevent disease and improve health. Thereby increasing their recovery from illness and assuming control of their own health. Kenneth Cohen in his entertaining and informative book, 'The Way of Qigong (Ch'i Kung): The Art and Science of Chinese Energy Healing', uses your ability to manage your money as an example of how be successful when cultivating ch'i. 'Success requires competence in accumulating, maintaining, and replenishing your 'principal'.

The language of ancient Israel was Hebrew, one of the Semitic languages of the Middle East. It is the language in which most of the Hebrew Bible, what Christians call the Old Testament, was originally written. Literature in Hebrew has been produced continuously since at least the 12th century BC. It is written that God breathed into the Earth to create the first human being, and the breath of God is synonymous with the power of the human spirit.

> And god formed man of the dust of the ground, and breathed into his nostrils the breath of life; and man became a living soul.
>
> *The Bible, Genesis 2:7*

Islam and its holy book the Qur'an, compiled around 651AD expresses similar beliefs; the followers of Islam, Muslims, believe that God revealed the contents of the Qur'an to Muhammad through the angel Gabriel. The Holy Scripture was revealed to Muhammad in Arabic and provided the people of that time with a holy book, which is today considered as one of the finest examples of classical Arabic prose. In the Qur'an, Allah speaking to angels, 'I am going to create man from dried clay...so when I have fashioned him completely and breathed into him the soul which I created for him...' Shaykh Hakim Moinuddin Chishti, in his book *The Book of Sufi Healing*, explains that 'breath' is not the same as air or oxygen; it is a celestial energy that is a hub for your emotions and determines your balanced state, where 'Both the quantity and quality of breath have a definite and direct effect upon human health.'

Anaximenes, a Greek philosopher living in 545BC, declared that air is the source of all matter and all life started with a breath. All things come from it and dissolve into it at death. The soul is the breath that controls and holds together human beings. His major contribution, however, was stating that nothing could be created from nothing. Matter, force, and energy are indestructible. These ideas later reappeared in physics in the laws of the conservation of matter and energy.

Long before the Europeans discovered America, the inhabitants of the Americas were the American Indians. Modern cities now dominate areas, which were once their communities filled with minimal structures and languages of finite details. The American Indians would talk of the sacred breath as a healing force, and use chants and breathing methods to drive away disease and illness. The Sioux American Indian tribes believed that the strength and spirit of a man was in his breath. They viewed the spirit of a man as immortal, and that it was breathed into him by the 'great mystery', which ultimately returned to the source once it was released upon death.

The native Australian people, Aborigines, a name derived from the Latin phrase *ab origine*, meaning 'from the beginning'. For centuries without a written language, and long before any other people arrived, they had created songs and stories that encompassed their beliefs. They believed that their 'Yowee bulleerul', the Aborigine for 'spirit breath', was an innate connection between their body and spirit.

The Samurai of early Asia talk of the harmony of breathing, as being the harmony of mind. They believed that control of their breathing would give them the power and energy for mental focus and concentration. In Kaiten Nukariyan's book, The Religion of the Samurai, this belief is expressed poetically:

> Compressing his breathings let him, who has subdued all
> motions, breathe forth through the nose with the gentle
> breath. Let the wise man without fail restrain his mind,
> that chariot yoked with vicious horses.

Oxygen: The good, the bad, and the ugly
The good
It is stating the obvious when it is said that oxygen is vital for life. Nevertheless, in some ways this obvious human need deflects attention away from the real issues such as the quality of your breathing and the performance of your respiratory system. These two factors will greatly affect your health and well-being, as they form the basis of how your body creates, protects and sustains your life. Oxygen is critical in

maintaining your homeostasis (a balanced body) and generates the majority of energy required to power your activities, thoughts, feelings, and actions.

The bad
Part I - Unnatural breathing attacks your health
Professor of Psychology at Hunter College, New York, Robert Fried, Ph.D., in his research in to the psychology and physiology of breathing, analysed the effects of chronic rapid breathing called 'the hyperventilation syndrome'. This unnatural breathing, or to use a more visual term 'chest breathing' was proven to be inefficient. It is characterised by increased breathing rates, irregular or interrupted breathing, and frequent sighing. Breathing that uses the chest instead of the diaphragm does not allow as much air into your lungs. To compensate, the breathing rate increases to ensure the same amount of air going in and out of the lungs each minute, mimicking the symptoms of the hyperventilation syndrome. In patients with airflow obstruction (e.g. asthma), hyperinflation of lungs, stretches lung tissue, and leads to additional elastic recoil, forcing a portion of the diaphragm downward and a shortening of muscle fibres.

Emotional situations and unhealthy stress can also cause distress to your breathing efficiency, and will result in the same effects as hyperventilation. Hyperventilation causes a detrimental effect to the chemistry of the blood. The blood loses carbon dioxide at a higher rate and these losses in turn cause an increase in the blood alkaline levels. Even though there is plenty of oxygen in the blood, the alkaline shift in the blood interferes with the oxygen-releasing blood cells, which leads to less oxygen being delivered to the cells. This reduction of usable oxygen in the system resulted in reduced energy and the impaired ability to perform basic metabolic functions. Furthermore, it was observed that the reductions in usable oxygen blood flow could be contributing factors to heart disease, increased blood pressure, and stroke. It found that it may also contribute to some migraines, anxiety and epileptic attacks. In addition, as the body reacts to try to redress the body balance, increased stress, nervousness, tension, overexcitement could increase the prevalence of headaches, ulcers, and muscular pains.

Dr Fried went on to talk about the 'breath connection' concerning many diseases that blight the lives of people everyday. It is seen as a symptom in many diseases. People are being increasingly deprived of precious oxygen in the modern environment, and it is causing serious health problems as numerous studies and research on oxygen deficiency have shown. Starvation at the cellular level causes cells to be too weak to manufacture the enzymes that protect them, and the oxygen-starved cells are vulnerable to virus and pathogen attack.

Medical symptoms of oxygen deficiency include: acid stomach, bacterial, viral and parasitic infections, bronchial problems, chronic hostility, circulation problems, depression, dizziness, fatigue, irrational behaviour, irritation, lowered immunity to colds, flu and infections, memory loss, muscle aches, overall body weakness, poor digestion, tumours and deposit build-ups. These medical symptoms often begin with a vague feeling of uneasiness. They progress over time, to full-blown illness and disease. Cells undergoing partial oxygen starvation send out tiny panic signals that are collectively felt as a continuous vague sensation of uneasiness, dread, or disaster. This low-level generalized warning tends to be turned out as mere background noise by the individual experiencing it. Alternatively, it is attributed to other sources of uneasiness.

Irregular rapid breathing is measured around 18 plus breaths per minute (normal breathing is 12 per minute); at this level anxiety is aggravated and could progress onto panic disorders at 30 breaths per minute. Ultimately, under severe stress your breathing rate can rise to, as much as 100 breaths per minute! It is estimated that 135 million Americans suffer from hyperventilation, which is complex and multifaceted in origin, and a symptom of many diseases. Dr Fried points out that addressing the 'breath connection' may have a part to play in the treatments of diseases, and his observations recorded that correct breathing can reverse the effects of hyperventilation, and enhance the blood flow to the brain.

The bad
Part II - Oxygen Deficiency Disease
Oxygen deficiency in a person's body tissue is a sure indicator for disease. Hypoxia, shortages of oxygen in body tissue, is the fundamental cause for all degenerative diseases.

> Insufficient oxygen means insufficient biological energy that can result in anything from mild fatigue to life threatening disease. The connection between insufficient oxygen and disease has now been firmly established.
>
> *Dr Way*
> *Journal of the American Association of Physicians*

Inadequate supplies in your oxygen levels will damage your ability to sustain maximum health, vitality, a boosted immune system, and successful aging. The evidence suggests that humans are meant to function with higher concentrations of oxygen in their systems. Lower oxygen levels leads to poor health, lower energy levels, and inefficient metabolism. This inefficient system leads to the accumulation of disease contributing toxins, which would ordinarily be burned in normal metabolic functioning. Ultimately, it leads to chronic illness and disease.

Dr Warburg, the two-time Nobel Prize winner for cancer research, explains that the lack of oxygen plays a major role in causing cells to become cancerous, as the normal oxygen respiration cells are replaced by anaerobic (without oxygen) cell respiration.

The ugly

The body creates energy to live, and in the process produces oxidants (or free radicals), which when produced in excess quantities can be harmful to health. The harmful pressure the body is placed under by the free radicals is referred to as oxidising stress. Problems start to occur when the free radical production exceeds the body's ability to protect against them.

> It is a relatively simple matter to turn a stable molecule or compound into the free radical species simply by bringing it in contact with another free radical...The whole exchange takes microseconds. Once a free radical is present it tends to propagate by generating other free radicals from chain reactions....
>
> *Leslie Kenton*
> Author of *Age Power*

The causes of this oxidising stress are numerous and varied. Some people take in more than others, like the archaic smoker, who inhales in just one puff, a trillion of these 'uglies' in one go. Eating foods that create excessive blood sugar swings and poor insulin controls (like consumption of high sugar refined foods) will cause oxidation damage. Transportation fumes, pollution, oil burning, and over exposure to the sun will all contribute to the unleashing of the free radicals.

Leslie Kenton, in her groundbreaking book *Age Power*, identifies six of the harmful effects caused by the free radicals and oxidising stress. She points out that oxidising stress will damage your cells' DNA, which affects and inhibits the ability of the cells to experience energy; it exposes the brain and nervous system to poison (toxicity); and there is a dysfunction in the cell mitochondria (your energy producers and calorie-burning machines). In addition, goes on to add that these free radicals can also damage cell membranes that cause cell malnourishment, damage to your body's protein, and weaken your immune system. The collective detrimental effect of this oxidising stress means that a person can suffer problems such as energy deficiency, increased risks of illness and disease, greater levels of body fat, higher incidents of stress, reduction in brain cells, and premature aging (for instance, more wrinkles than you should have).

The cavalry
In the face of the terrorising free radicals and the damage they can unleash on your life, there is a need for personal protection; your body can call on the protective force of the antioxidants. The antioxidants have the power to protect and in some cases reverse the effects of the oxidants. There is an army of nutrients whose deployment is in your hands, with a little help from the enzyme released by the body. These are nutrients such as vitamin A, C, E and D, beta-carotene, minerals selenium, and zinc, as well as plant superhero's phytonutrients and flavonoids. All you have to do is consume them (as part of a real food nutritional plan), to fight back and reclaim your health and well-being. In Part three - Nourishment you will find details on how to discover and utilise these nutrients to reclaim your vitality and health.

The last lung of defence
The lungs are the most fragile organ in the body, and it is vital that you protect them whenever possible, otherwise debilitating conditions such as asthma, chronic obstructive pulmonary disease (COPD), lung fibrosis, lung cancer or mesothelioma can develop. Risks of injury originate from the inhalation of particles, gases, or fumes. It is the size of these particles, which determines how far they penetrate the lungs, which has a three-layered defence structure:

> **Defence No.1**: The lungs have a protective waste removal escalator and clears (coughed or swallowed) approximately 90% of particles within two hours. This speed of clearance can be affected by toxic fumes, severe air pollution, and exposure to cigarette smoke.

> **Defence No.2**: The alveolar defence are the macrophages, and are residents of the body cells; they kill non-living particles or alien bacteria, and then leave enzymes to do the clearing up.

> **Defence No.3**: The lymphatic drainage transport system is a 'flushing' system, where lymphatic fluid, and any particles, from the left and right lungs are flushed out.

Will these defences be able to cope with the increasing pollution attacks?

Chapter 2

Pollution protection

There is an insatiable desire to raise the standards of living throughout the world; this desire, knowingly or unknowingly, leaves behind a trail of consumption which results in high levels of pollution, contaminating the environment.

Earth has had to endure incidents of chemical waste contamination where the land, water, and air have been rendered virtually uninhabitable. People unfortunate enough to be in, or close to, those contaminated areas are shown to have increased risks of illness, disease, and higher mortality rates.

All living things exert some pressure on the environment. The extent of environmental pollution caused by humans is already so great that some scientists question whether the Earth can continue to support life unless immediate corrective action is taken.

> 'We should all be concerned about the future because we
> will have to spend the rest of our lives there'.
>
> *Charles F. Kettering*

Ecology and environmental deterioration

Earth supports some five million species of plants, animals, and microorganisms. These interact and influence their surroundings, and form a vast network of interrelated environmental systems called ecosystems. The arctic tundra is an ecosystem, so is a Brazilian rain forest, and the islands of Hawaii are a relatively isolated ones. If left undisturbed, natural environmental systems will achieve balance and stability among its various species of plants and animals. Complex ecosystems can also compensate for changes caused by weather or intrusions from migrating animals, and are more stable than the simple ecosystems. The effects of human activities are not so easy to compensate for, as their activities have caused the extinction of a number of plant and animal species, while endangering others.

Population Explosion

The reduction of the Earth's resources has been closely linked to the rise in human population. In the 19th century, the Industrial Revolution placed greater pressures on the environment, by effecting a dramatically increased population and an amplified level of pollution. Although industrial development improved the standard of living, there was a great environmental cost. The Earth was home to 6.5 billion people at the beginning of the 21st century - twice the total in 1960 and is projected to reach a staggering 9.1 billion by 2050. The human population boom is located and increasingly concentrated in large urban areas, where 80% of people live.

In addition, an important factor alongside population is the rates of human consumption. For example, North America consumes fifteen times more energy than the continent of Africa. Populations are the driving force behind consumption with the increases in income, nutrition, energy needs, and global markets.

In 1952, thousands of people died in severe pollution episodes; over 5,000 in one week alone were killed in London. In the decades since then, the air pollution problems for developed and emerging countries had centred on the combustion by-products arising from the use of coal, both domestic and industrial. Although in recent times the primary pollution concerns for developed and emerging countries have been diverted elsewhere, the poorer countries of the world continue to suffer from the effects of burning coal, which continue to cause premature deaths in predominantly women and children.

Outdoor pollution

The negative influences of air pollution affect people in varied, complex, and intricate ways. Lungs are exposed daily to dangerous elements such as dust, traffic fumes, and factory and power station smoke, which are very harmful when inhaled. Around 24,000 people die prematurely each year due to outdoor pollution in the United Kingdom, and it unfairly discriminates against people with a pre-existing lung condition, such as children, and the elderly.

The underground transport systems carry a very high risk of air pollution. In October 2001, scientists from the University College London warned that air quality in carriages and at stations were up to 73 times worse than at street level. So much so that, it is suggested that travelling for twenty minutes on a tube train through central London had the same effect on the lungs as smoking a cigarette.

The numbers of pollutants, which have known or suspected harmful effects to human health or the environment, are increasing as the scientists conduct further investigations and experiments. Different areas in the world have differing pollution concerns. In the industrialised blocks of Europe the pollutants are principally products of combustion, power stations, transportation (car, trucks, trains, aeroplanes etc.), and heating (of buildings, and space). The resulting pollutants, such as ozone, airborne particles, and nitrogen dioxide cause many people to suffer from a variety of illnesses and diseases. In addition, existing sufferers of illnesses or diseases such as asthma, respiratory, and cardiovascular, endure conditions made worse, and sometimes fatal, by the ongoing exposure to these resultant pollutants. At high pollution levels, even the healthiest person is susceptible to breathing difficulties.

> Young and healthy highway patrol officers were the subject of research headed by Michael Riediker of the Institute of Occupational Health Sciences, Switzerland, into the harmful effects of exposure to traffic emissions. The results showed worrying interference with the heart functions, causing irregular beats, and eliciting inflammatory and thrombotic responses.

> In a further study reviewing thirty-five plus studies of workers with occupational exposure to diesel exhaust, it was shown that the excess risk of lung cancer was consistently elevated by 20 to 50%.

> Furthermore, a 38-year study of 54,973 U.S. railroad workers, who worked on diesel-powered trains, showed similar results of elevated lung cancer risks. However, much more interestingly, they concluded that 'there was no relationship between years of exposure and [the] lung cancer risk'. Their lung mortality risk did not increase with increasing years of work. Therefore, it can be concluded that any duration of exposure can result in an elevated risk.

Today, traffic emissions have taken over as the biggest threat to your health and environment. The primary threats are carbon monoxide, nitrogen oxides, and volatile organic compounds, which are released into the air every time a petrol or diesel powered motor vehicle is used. This then starts a chain reaction, where photochemical interactions release a secondary, long-range pollutant into the air, often miles from the original emission site. Ozone is formed when sunlight reacts with nitrogen dioxide and the volatile organic compounds. The nitrogen oxides greatly influence another long-range pollutant, acid rain.

The long-rangers
You do not even have to be in the immediate vicinity to be exposed to these pollutants, as they can travel long distances, and by chemically

reacting along the way, can produce secondary pollutants such as acid rain or ozone. In all except worst-case situations, industrial and domestic pollutant sources, together with their impact on air quality, tend to be steady state or improving over time. However, traffic pollution problems are worsening worldwide. The Keck School of Medicine at the University of Southern California using data from two clinical trials involving 798 participants, showed in the first published research providing epidemiologic evidence, that there was a clear association between atherosclerosis (coronary artery disease) and ambient air pollution.

Heavy traffic ahead
Richard Dahl's 'Heavy Traffic Ahead: Car Culture Accelerates' details the growing concerns of the increasing use of vehicles globally, and highlights China, the world's biggest nation, and its role in the issue of the increasing traffic problem.

China's rate of car ownership is low by the standards of the developed world, but it is increasing at a very fast rate. Between the late 1970's and 2001, China's overall fleet of motor vehicles (excluding two wheeled ones) increased ten-fold. Along the way, the Chinese government decided it wanted to develop its own auto industry. In 2001, China identified auto manufacturing as one of seven "pillar industries" of the Chinese economy and announced a five-year plan to implement a primarily domestic industry that could offer a Chinese family car at a price that would encourage widespread ownership. Between 2000 and 2004, production of passenger cars in China jumped from 605,000 to 2.33 million. On 5th February 2005, the China Federation of Machinery Industry, forecast 20% growth for 2005 to a level that would move China past Germany into third place globally for motor vehicle production. Most industry analysts believe that the industry will continue to expand in the 15% range annually for years to come.

The government has also encouraged private investments in highways to fuel a road-building program, which is already well under way to accommodate the growing number of vehicles. In October 2004, China's Ministry of Communication announced that the nation's freeways had reached 30,000 kilometres, placing it behind only the United States. The attention is focused on China, and with due concern, but people who follow international transportation issues say the trend in motorisation is global.

The fastest growth is occurring in Asia and Latin America, and the number of motor vehicles (excluding two wheeled ones) in the world is expected to double in the next fifteen years to 1.3 billion. Increasing numbers of vehicles of all types in developing countries will result in further deteriorating air quality, greater congestion, and poorer quality of life. There will be increases in air pollutants carbon monoxide, nitrogen oxide, and ozone, with the carbon dioxide emissions alone in excess of fourteen billion per year.

What can you do to help?

On the road

- Use public transport whenever you can
- Avoid using your car for short journeys - 2.5 km (~1.5 miles) or less
- If possible, don't use your car at all during periods of high pollution
- Start your engine only once you are ready to move off
- Don't rev the engine unnecessarily
- Drive smoothly. Heavy braking and rapid acceleration means you use more fuel and increase pollution
- Keep to the speed limit
- Maintain your car. Keep the engine properly tuned and the tyres at the right pressure
- Reduce ownership to one per household

It's Showtime

An investigation carried out by reporters for the Guardian, a UK newspaper revealed that the Chinese government with its authoritarian methods is seeking to engineer 'blue skies' over the city of Beijing during the 2008 Olympic Games. For the duration of the games, they will place driving bans on two million cars, stop work on thousands of building sites, and shutdown power plants and factories. Then call on scientific intervention, and spray the roads and skies with chemicals to induce precipitation, and reduce the particle air matter.

The chances of success are stacked against them, and the worst set of recorded data in recent years proves it. In 2006, severe pollution affected 65% of the days for January, and if this trend were to continue, would mean that before the end of April they will have already surpassed the recorded number of severely polluted days for the whole of 2005.

The pollution effect on women

A growing bulk of evidence links chronic exposure to air pollution with increased risks of mortality (due to diseases such as heart, lung, and respiratory). A new study corroborates this evidence, and highlights the fact that women may be at greater risks of fatal coronary heart disease than men, due to the exposure to airborne particle-matter. Moreover, when ozone or sulphur dioxide is also present, the risk to women is even greater.

The study, by a team of epidemiologists at Loma Linda University, is part of the 22-year Adventist Health Study on the Health Effects of Smog. The study followed 3,239 female non-smokers, mainly in urban areas of California from 1976 to 1998, and led the researchers to conclude that there was '…an elevated risk of fatal CHD [coronary heart disease] associated with ambient levels of [particle matter]…'

Women were again at the centre of a study by the University of Düsseldorf, where over 4,000 women between 1985 and 1994 showed a higher risk of developing chronic obstructive pulmonary disease, and suffering detrimental effects on lung function from air pollution if they resided close to busy roads.

Pregnancy births are also adversely affected by the exposure to air pollution. Analyses conducted by the University of California for women living in Los Angeles, covering the period 1989 to 2000, showed that women residing in high pollution areas, were up to 36% at a greater risk of their baby reporting a low birth weight and at a 30% increased risk of a preterm birth.

The health risks of smoking weigh heavier on women living in the United States than other women around the world. For instance, they contribute only 5% to the total of world smokers but a substantial 50% to the total of those who die from smoking related diseases.

Indoor air pollution

The World Health Organisation report on 'Indoor air pollution and health' claimed that 'in poorly ventilated dwellings, indoor smoke can exceed acceptable levels for small particles in outdoor air a hundred-fold. Exposure is particularly high among women and children, who spend the most time near the domestic hearth. Every year, indoor air pollution is responsible for the death of 1.6 million people, that is one death every 20 seconds'.

Your homes and workplaces, due to the nature of the confined space, represent higher risks of lung irritation. Tobacco smoke, animal fur and dusts, mould, mildew and bacteria, house dust mites, cooking and heating appliances, and asbestos have all proved to be harmful to human health, coupled with other dangerous substances such as formaldehyde gas, and toxic chemicals found in some household cleaning products, paints, solvents, and pesticides, can make the home a very hostile environment.

What can you do to help?
- Use water-based or low-solvent products - paints, glues, varnishes, wood preservatives, etc.

- Reduce your central heating temperature by a few degrees
- In the garden avoid burning household waste, especially plastics and rubber
- If you have to BBQ, use gas powered appliances

Home: haven or harbour

Battelle, an organisation specialising in future trend predictions, recently identified what it believes to be the healthy trends of the future home. The forecast listed ten trends likely to occur before 2010, and among the ten were 'Breathing easy: Indoor air quality' and 'Mite wars'. Battelle suggests that in the years to come households will seek more products and services to increase air ventilation and filtration, and decrease the humidity, mould, and indoor air pollutants. Some of these type products or services are available today, but these are usually marketed and sold to those existing sufferers of respiratory diseases and allergies. Battelle suggest that in the years to come these type products will be aimed at every household or business; to the point where a future home will be sold with such products included as standard.

> The impact of housing on health and safety has emerged as a major public health concern. The whole basis for the initiative was to encourage public health programs to address multiple housing deficiencies and hazards that affect the health and safety of residents.
>
> *Jerry Hershovitz*
> *National Center for Environmental Health*

Modern homes, with their added insulation and double-glazing, can trap contaminants inside, producing a cocktail of odours, fumes, and tiny creatures. One of these dangers are 'mites', which are devilish tiny insects that are found in bedrooms or similar places that are warm and dark. They are very difficult to eliminate and are said to be responsible for numerous different allergies. When air pollutants are trapped inside a home, office, room, or space, it can magnify, by up to 500 times the adverse health effects caused. Spending large amounts of time in such places can lead to symptoms such as headaches, eye, nose, and throat irritation; a dry cough; dry or itchy skin; dizziness and nausea; difficulty in concentrating; fatigue; and sensitivity to odours.

How to improve your living or working space:

- Increasing the ventilation and air circulation is often the best means of reducing indoor pollutant levels. Kitchen, bathroom and garages, are strong pollutant sources, and air should be vented directly to the outside

- Reduce the reliance on heating and air-conditioning units; if you have to use them then service them regularly
- Replace or renovate areas of water damage such as mould, damp, and leakages immediately
- Ensure effective pest control
- Decrease use and storage of aerosols, toxic paints, solvents, pesticides, and adhesives
- Do not allow anyone to smoke in your home
- Limit the time pets are indoors
- Remove dust and dirt daily
- Air purifiers are an option but have (at the moment) have a limited coverage and success

Where there is smoke, there is lung cancer

Smoking is the leading preventable cause of premature death from heart disease, lung cancer, and cancer. In the USA and UK, 65 million people are regular smokers and each year over 530,000 die of premature illness due to smoking. Chronic cigarette smokers will live on average 18 years less than non-smokers and each cigarette smoked provides 4,000 plus toxins that shortens life by at least seven minutes! According to a recent survey by the World Health Organisation, three million people die each year of smoking related illnesses. By 2020, the death toll will rise to an estimated ten million per year, and of the people alive today, tobacco will contribute to ten billion deaths.

- Stop today for immediate benefits
- 24 hrs – Lungs start to clear themselves of mucus
- 72 hrs – Cough and breathing start to ease
- 2.5 years – Lung cancer risk reduced by 50%
- 3 to 5 years – Heart attack risks similar to non-smoker
- 5 to 10 years – Risks of major health problems similar to people who have never smoked

Passive smoking, the breathing of other peoples cigarette smoke, is estimated in the UK alone, to hospitalise 17,000 under five-year-olds, and cause the deaths of 1,000. A non-smoker, living or working in a smoke-filled environment over a prolonged period, increases their risk of lung cancer by a third. Governments are tackling this problem by passing legislation that will, or which has already done so, outlaw smoking in public places. As a result, many restaurants, cinemas, transport facilities such as airlines and trains, and offices are smoke-free. However, as long as Governments receive large tax revenues from tobacco products, and manufacturers and distributors continue to make good profits off the back of the addictive substance, then it is unlikely the a total ban of the human poison will ever occur.

A European example of smoking action...and inaction
The European Union has banned tobacco advertising in print media, on the radio and internet, and at cross-border events or activities. European Member states had until July 2005 to introduce the legislation into national law. While most countries have adopted the common-sense measures, and implemented the ban, others cannot see through the haze of smoke. In April 2006, the Reuters agency for Berlin reported that the European Commission was taking legal action against four countries for not enforcing the ban, and another two countries for not introducing the legislation into national law.

Respiratory diseases (as well as disorders, such as allergic rhinitis, atopic eczema, and urticaria) have shown considerable global increases in both prevalence and severity since the 1960's. The rises of prevalence have occurred in both children and adults. Because this rise has been far too rapid to implicate any genetic basis for change, it has been attributed to environmental and lifestyle factors. Asthma is one of these diseases and is a major long-term respiratory disorder in the United Kingdom (UK). About 3.7 million adults and 1.4 million children are currently receiving treatment for asthma, costing the UK health service £2.3 billion.

In the UK, disease affected people are being overlooked due to Government financial and strategic pressures, and means that millions of people live with a lottery for a health service. This health service lottery is dependant on what your disease is, the facilities you use, and its cost. For instance, those who suffer lung disease can be seen as less important than other illnesses. Over the period 2000 to 2005, the numbers hospitalised were extremely high and unchanging. The hospital admission costs alone are £1.08 billion, and the knock-on effect is that twenty-five million workdays are lost with a financial cost to businesses estimated at £1.5 billion. However, the amount of money spent on research into the various lung diseases has gone down since the year 1999.The Medical Research Council only spends 3.8 per cent of their gross expenditure on respiratory research. Of all the monies spent on cancer research only three per cent is spent on lung cancer where over 35,000 people die each year from the disease. The treatment of lung cancer in the UK puts them at the bottom of the European league of lung cancer morbidity.

Working towards disease
Lung diseases caused by asbestos exposure (called mesothelioma) increased by 56% between the years 1989 and 1999. According to the

British Lung Foundation, a new group of people are affected by mesothelioma. Occupations recorded on death certificates from recent deaths indicate that building workers, especially plumbers, gas fitters, carpenters, and electricians are now the largest high-risk occupational groups. Many other people (normally those with lower socioeconomic status and thus less choice in how they earn a living) are putting their lives at risk in order to satisfy, ultimately, the consumer. These practices go on without scrutiny and thousands of deaths recorded without outcry.

In China, and in numerous other countries, the international jewellery trade is the culprit of such instances. In one area of China, Guangdong, there are 2,000 factories accounting for £1.5 billion and 50% of the country's gems like onyx, quartz, and crystal, in order to keep up with the demand from the international jewellery markets in the United States and Europe. Workers in some of these factories work without facemasks in inadequately ventilated rooms. The ultra fine particles are inhaled and can result in silicosis, a disease of the lungs, which take about eight years for the symptoms to appear, in which time they suffer coughing fits and acute difficulties in breathing. Ultimately, their lungs will fail. According to the Chinese Health Ministry, some 440,000 work related lung disease deaths (although experts question the figure as being an extremely low estimate) occurred in China. This 'silicosis epidemic' led one United Kingdom national newspaper, The Sunday Times, to run an exposé story the 'Deadly dust of the gem trade kills Chinese'.

One of the companies involved was Perfect Gem & Pearl Manufacturing. When confronted by the investigators a bullish company spokesperson retorted 'Our Company has spent a lot of money to improve ventilation and equipment. There are about six hundred workers in the factory now. If the working conditions are really bad, why are they still here?' The jewellery industry reputation is threatened by such investigations and when hard-pressed into action, and for a response to such allegations, the World Jewellery Confederation issued a limp and worthless call on 'foreign buyers to investigate the epidemic, to press for compensation and to lobby for better conditions'. Is it really the role of buyers to investigate such allegations or lobby for better conditions? While token and toothless confederations and associations like this one exist, then it is undoubtedly a role for buyers and consumers. By refusing to purchase such unethical products, the consumer can deliver the most powerful message of all.

The future pollutants
Scientists worldwide are continuing to discover unique properties of everyday materials at the most minuscule scale. Nanoparticles, a

billionth the size of a particle, are one such area, of which you are going to hear a lot more about. These particles have already been transposed to the commercial market in the shape of products like sunscreens, toothpastes, and even some food products! The nanoparticles are also to be found in plastic fillers, car tyres, and continuing to find uses within the biological field. The scientists enthusiastically hail nanoparticles as the 'next big thing' with massive potential to change lives. They trumpet the benefits to both the consumer and industry as they plough worldwide investments into its science.

However, there are opponents to this technology and research is beginning to surface regarding the potentially harmful effects of these particles if they enter the human body. Entry is possible through the lungs and has the potential to translocate to the blood, and thereby reach other targets such as the cardiovascular system, spleen, liver, and the brain. The nanoparticles once inside the body have been shown to affect and interfere with the body cells. A substantial literature demonstrates that these pose a hazard to the lungs through their potential to cause oxidative stress, inflammation, and cancer; they also have the potential to redistribute to other organs following pulmonary deposition. There is no universal "nanoparticle", and each nanomaterial has to be treated individually when health risks are expected. Nanoparticles therefore, can be seen as a group of particulate toxins with abilities to cause injury, and with dangerous translocation properties, which have the potential to mediate a range of adverse effects in the lungs and other organs.

These nanoparticles can be designed for drug delivery or as food components, and it will need strong legislation and industry policing to investigate the potentially lethal health implications. Who has the strength to stand in the way of the commercial bulldozer or the money to investigate the potential adverse health implications?

Chapter 3

Rejuvenate inside-out

In this chapter, you will discover ways in which you can make a difference and start to enjoy a new lease of life. Using breathing activities you will improve the way you breathe, create a more efficient and empowering process, and enjoy benefits such as increased energy, vitality, and mental focus; reduced stress levels; strengthened immune system; renewed body parts and invigorated functions; reversed premature aging.

The average adult will breathe around twelve times per minute. There is no perfect number for you or me. However, you can achieve many benefits by proactively lowering that number from where it is now. The time, location, and your mood are all factors, which can affect your breaths per minute. The more stressed you are the more rapid and inefficient, your breathing becomes. Indeed your breathing rate is an excellent indicator of the emotional state of your body. Through breathing practices and awareness, you will be able to gain control over debilitating mood swings and negative stresses. Remember, it is not your goal to restrict or artificially control your breathing, but merely to exact awareness of it and in doing so return the process to its natural course.

Breathing deep
If a person was asked to 'take a deep breath', for most people this is what it would look like for the observer. First there is an audible intake of air, simultaneously the upper chest expands and the shoulders rise, followed by a holding of the breath (for about three to five seconds), a louder noise on exhalation, and a collapsing of the chest and shoulders. For one reason or another, people are inaccurately conditioned into thinking that a 'deep' breath, is one like that. When was the last time you were sat down and coached on how to breathe? Is there really a need to 'learn' how to breathe?

Take a closer look at your normal breathing process by identifying your breathing characteristics on the next page:

(Circle the one/s applicable)

I breathe through the:	mouth	nose

On **inhalation**, I detect movement in my:

chest	abdomen	shoulders

The movement is:	upward	outward

On **exhalation**, I detect movement in my:

chest	abdomen	shoulders

The movement is:	downward	inward

My breathing is:

noisy	audible	silent	wheezy

My breath feels like it is: *(Circle all that apply)*

choppy	smooth	shallow	fast
light	heavy	irregular	easy
distressed	even	intense	forced
deep	random	disrupted	rushed

During infancy, your breathing works on an automatic pilot allowing for little interference, and the breathing is as close to perfect as you can get. However, it is not long before children are able to interfere with their 'perfect' breathing patterns such as throwing temper tantrums or overreacting. When confronted with stressful or emotional situations it is common to hear someone to say something like 'take a deep breath' in an attempt to calm the situation. If used, as it should be, then these words are truly wise ones. When you hear the words 'take a deep breath', it is not an instruction to take in as much volume of air as you can or hold it for an abnormal length of time. It is an instruction to draw your attention to the quality, rate, and depth of the breathing. By increasing the quality of your breathing by reducing the rate (to normal), and lowering the body movement to the abdomen, and not the chest area, you will have discovered the active forces enabling you to calm your emotions at any given instance.

The way of natural breathing

Most adults breathe best when asleep, and if it were replicated during the day, it would enhance life in measurable and dramatic ways. Imagine your day, starting and finishing with the same heightened energy level, conducting your daily activities with added zest and vitality, and having an alert and calm disposition. The way of natural breathing, aims to take those mental images and make them real.

Simplicity makes the way of natural breathing its most favourable attribute and biggest attraction. Dr Vogel, the author of The Nature Cure, recounts some amazing body and health adaptations after discovering breathing activities. He enthusiastically reported improved sleep, and decreased levels of stress and anxiety. His digestion had improved, and the stomach pain and inflammation, which plagued him for weeks, had disappeared. Dr Vogel goes on to explain how correct breathing influences illness and disease, and lists the many areas that are positively affected by correct breathing such as the nervous system, conditions such as angina, asthma, bronchitis, constipation, abdominal complaints, and weight management (claiming that you can lose weight and reports a 50% success rate). In fact, he goes on to say 'Indeed, no illness or disease exists that will not benefit from correct breathing techniques'.

The Nature Cure (Der kleine Doktor – the German title) was first published in 1952, is in its 50th plus edition, and sold millions of copies worldwide. He practised what he preached and lived to the golden age of 94.

The breathing cycle

To reiterate, the process of breathing is identified by the four distinct stages: 1.The inhalation of air; 2.The crossover stage and exchange of gases; 3.Exhalation, and 4.The natural pause before the next inhalation (and the restart of the process).

Firstly, it is important that you actually identify the four stages while you breathe. Awareness of the four stages is an enlightening and empowering one. The cycle begins as you:

- **Inhale through your nose**
  Your tongue should hug the roof of your closed mouth
  Push your abdomen out as you inhale

The nose is the royal red carpet of the breathing process, it welcomes and warms the air on the inhalation, and on its finely groomed hairs it traps dust, pollutants and germs, that will be cleared out later on. It is the body's preferred option and should be yours. Focus on the air as it enters the channels of the nose; you should feel the sensation of the air passing over the fine nose hairs. Onward down the back of your throat, and deep into your lungs. Place your hands on or around your belly button to feel the air push outward. There should be no lifting or expanding of the chest or upward shoulder movement.

- **Allow for the exchange of oxygen / carbon dioxide**

The gaseous exchange takes place. Do not try to elongate, extend, or alter this stage. Just try to acknowledge its existence.

- **Exhale through the nose**

With hands still on your abdomen, you should feel them move inwards in the direction of your backbone. Again, follow the journey of the air from the lungs, up the back of your throat and divided through your nose. The lung reflex should make this stage effortless.

- **The pause**

Again, just observe. There is a sense of immense power and weakness in the brief pause. It exudes the power to give life and the weakness of total dependency. It is a brief reflective pause, on which the body congratulates itself on the perfection of each breath cycle. It is a non-stopping, incessant cycle of waves, and like every other part of the body has an inbuilt mechanism for securing a period of rest. Albeit a very brief one, this pause is the moment of rest and relaxation of the breathing process. The faster you breathe the less opportunity for rest, and the greater the increase risks of malfunction and injury, leading eventually to an illness or disease.

Anytime awareness
You have the opportunity to exact the ability to change both your state of mind and body at anytime or place. The emotional rollercoaster and storing of stress (or disease deposits), can be resigned to history. You could be standing in a line of never-ending people, sitting in traffic, riding a packed train, or just 'enjoying' family life, these types of frustrating situations are numerous, and the accumulation of these stressors weigh heavily on your well-being. Finding yourself in these kinds of trying situations only requires a quick check on your breathing patterns to bring you back to natural alignment and allow you to maintain serenity and calmness. Its simplicity is the key; anytime, anywhere, and it works.

In the next chapter, Air space (and in more depth in Part four – R&R) you will find more detailed techniques to assist you and how to create more 'MeTo' opportunities to rejuvenate your body from the inside out.

Breathing activities explored
So far, you have developed an awareness of your natural breathing cycle, and now comes the time to discover activities to improve the efficiency of that cycle.

The breathing activities are best practiced in the morning as soon as you are awake or in your final preparations for when you sleep. Just one minute per day is enough to start with, to give you an energy boost and natural high. Simplicity again is the major asset for this activity. There is no need to count the breaths, or special positions to maintain, or prior preparations to make. Try the following activity, remembering to start with just one-minute.

■   Inhale through the nose; pushing the abdomen outward away from your backbone, with no movement in you chest or shoulders.

■   Exhale through the nose and pull in your abdomen. Keep the exhalation at a constant and even pace and the aim of the breathing activity is to pull in your stomach in as far as you possibly can. Imagine your belly button trying to reach your backbone.

Before you give it a try here are some helpful hints to help you perform this breathing activity:

- Try to keep all other aspects of the breathing cycle the same
- Ensure inhalation is similar to exhalation in length
- Increase or decrease the length of the activity according to your abilities to perform it
- Increase the length of time you practice until you reach the maximum of fifteen minutes per day
- An empty stomach is the most appropriate time to practise
- It is best performed lying down, standing, and in a seated body position

The more you practise the more chances are that you will see and feel the benefits of a more efficient breathing technique, and ultimately, a healthier you. It is a small investment of time, which will return exponentially higher rewards. You can look forward to

- improved and undisturbed sleep
- greater periods of relaxation
- higher levels of alertness and focus
- a proven way to manage your negative stress
- the ability to make a difference to your well-being
- improve you body functions, from lung capacity to digestion
- a natural 'instant mood and energy enhancer'

More breathing activities
It is time to explore further, the practical and colourful ways of using your newly found abilities to their maximum effect.

You will breathe 15,000 times a day, and a very impressive 5,475,000 (five million four hundred and seventy-five thousand) a year, give or take a few! In this breathing activity, you will need to find roughly thirty-six breaths (or three minutes) a day.

Rebalancing your body - part one – cleansing

The use of imagery to improve your breathing is a great way to channel your efforts and achieve what you want faster.

Instructions for Seated version:
Start as usual by increasing your awareness of your body's way of natural breathing. Focus on the four stages of the breathing cycle (observing but not interfering).

- Sitting comfortably with feet firmly on the floor, and hands placed on your thighs palms down. Close your eyes and you are ready to begin
- Imagine that gravity just got twice as powerful
- Your eyebrows and forehead feel heavier, and relax downward
- Your eyelashes and eyelids weigh a kilogram each; pupils weighted, your gaze is focused downward
- The weight of the ears sinks into the earlobes
- Relax your tongue off the roof of your mouth
- The jaw is relaxed and teeth are slightly parted
- Shoulders release all their tension, the arms sink deeper into your sides and backs of your hands into your thighs
- Fingers feel like they have added the weight of arms
- The blood circulates slower, and if you listen closely enough you can hear you heart pump
- Your legs feel like lead weights, bolted to the floor
- The feet and toes grow roots into the ground
- Allow the stresses, strains and pains, to flow out through your feet
- Release any control over your body, clearing out the harmful emotions and ills

This concludes the 'rebalancing your body' breathing activity, its aim is to bring your mind, and body to a place of perfect balance and by default ensures an optimum way of natural breathing. It is a two-part breathing activity, where the first part is the cleansing and rebalancing part, while the second is the rejuvenating and reenergising one.

Rebalancing your body – part two – rejuvenating

- Starting with the toes (left foot first), bring back the feeling and movement to them.
- Push your toes into the ground lifting the arch of the foot, so only, the toes and heels of your feet are touching the ground. Then again keeping the heels on the floor push the arches of the feet as flat to the ground as you can while lifting the toes into the air - Repeat this six times
- An electric current has now started its journey onwards and upwards, building in intensity and energy along the way
- Keeping the toes in contact with the ground, lift your heels as high as they can go (you should feel your calf muscles tighten) and then let fall back to the ground - Repeat 6 times
- From your seated position, swing both feet into the air and fully extend the legs, hold them there for a few seconds, and then place them on the floor - Repeat six times
- Squeeze and release the muscles of your abdomen and in your posterior - Repeat six times
- Starting with the little fingers make waves as though you were playing the piano, circle at the wrists first one way then the other – Repeat six times
- Lift the arms off the thighs and throw them up into the air, reaching as high as you can, first with one arm then the other. Keep pushing the fingertips higher and higher and then bring them back to a natural resting place - Repeat six times
- Lift your shoulders up trying to touch your earlobes and drop them lower then they normally rest - Repeat six times
- Repeat the arm and shoulder lifts again
- Open your mouth as wide as it can go lifting your eyebrows as well, and then bring it back into a smile as wide as you can - Repeat six times
- Stand up and reach into the air with both hands, then allow your arms to swing and sway in any direction.

This concludes the 'rejuvenating and reenergising' part of the breathing activity, its aim is to bring you back to life with a powerful energy. In Part four - R&R, you shall find out how you can use simple tools like this to renew and rejuvenate your life, and create unlimited amounts of energy and vitality.

Part two

Elixir of life

Water is a life inspiring and sustaining substance, and can be found in most living things. Humans are composed of around sixty percent of it; half of the brain is made up of it, muscle tissue holds seventy percent of it, and it contributes much to the body shape and structure. Water loss of any kind, for the human body will result in impaired functioning. Even, small losses in water will cause symptoms such as headaches, anger and irritability, forgetfulness, a lack of energy, and visual disturbances.

A period of days without water will start to affect the digestive, nervous, endocrine, cardiovascular, respiratory, waste elimination, thermo-regulatory, and reproductive systems, eventually leading to a partial shutdown of the body; if the period of water loss continues then it will be the cause of a person's death.

> It exists in the tree. It exists in the grass. It exists in the mountain. It exists in the river. It exists in the sea. It exists in the air. It exists in the cloud. Thus man is not only surrounded by water on all sides, but it penetrates his very body. But be can never appease his thirst without drinking water.
>
> *The religion of a samurai*

Throughout history, water has played a prominent part in the lives of people from ancient civilisations to modern man; it has determined where people choose to live, and has been the vital component of living such as, food production, power supply, cleansing, recreation, and worship. The access to clean water is being made more complicated and difficult each day and water pollution is now a prevalent part of modern life and the environment. Water is under attack from many sources such as inadequately treated sewage, fertilisers, silt, organic matter, petroleum, radioactive waste, heat, waste materials, pathogens, and pesticides. Coupled with extravagant usage and wastage, water shortages are now commonplace in a whole host of different countries and not just reserved for few countries in Africa. It cannot go on like this, and the once abundant and unlimited water supply, is most definitely an endangered one.

'Clean' water is your simple key to open a complex wealth of doors to deep and wondrous treasures. Treasures of rejuvenation, regeneration, an inner strength and resistance, a fluidity of thought and action, and a perpetual force of wellness are all yours for the taking; however, there is increasing need to fight for it, and you need to start today. In the following chapters you will discover how water can affect you, how to recognise the symptoms of dehydration which can occur on a daily basis. You will be provided with practical and effective advice on how to ensure that you have the optimum level of water in your system to guarantee the perfect foundations on which to build your good health, well-being, and youthfulness (as aging is partly a dehydration process). Your perfect hydration is as important as readjusting your lifestyle to reduce your pollution footprint on this Earth, and subsequently ensure the future of water for you and the generations to come.

Chapter 4

The wonders of water

A body not supplied with adequate water will start to fall below the optimum operating levels, and disrupt nutrient carrying fluids, digestion, toxic element excretion, temperature regulation, organ efficiency, and both mental and physical performance. In infants, children, and older adults the issue of dehydration is more serious and if not monitored and subsequently later addressed by qualified persons, it may result in their premature deaths.

If you are overweight with a high body fat ratio, you are at an even greater disadvantage. You will have a less effective temperature regulation mechanism, where your 'heating' mechanism (higher metabolic rate, excessive insulation, hormones, and thermal effects of eaten food) has a greater effect than your 'cooling' one (evaporation, convection, and conduction). This in turn has a greater impact on the physical and mental problems of inadequate water supplies.

The symptoms of an inadequate water supply for the average person include:

- recurrent headaches
- grogginess
- visual disturbances / irritations
- easily angered or irritable
- feeling exhausted
- hesitant and indecisive
- forgetfulness
- nervousness
- reduced capacity for mental or physical work
- digestive / bowel problems
- body temperature fluctuations

When we come to the individual needs for water, it is readily realized that water certainly is our most precious mineral. It is the most essential of all minerals for our bodies. An animal can lose all its fat, about half its protein, but if it loses as much as one-tenth of its water it will die.

Dr. Johnathan Forman

However, just flooding the body with as much water as you can will only produce unnecessary work for your kidneys, and increase the risks of other health complications. To restore balance, your kidneys release the excess water by excreting high-volume dilute urine. This can be dangerous and is referred to as 'water intoxication'. When water content is high in the body and your internal fluid pressure low, water is drawn into cells causing them to swell (which could pose an additional potential danger to brain cells).

Balancing act

The body has a fantastic way of ensuring the water content of the body remains, more or less, balanced over time. Briefly, the hypothalamus (part of the brain) produces antidiuretic hormone carried to the posterior pituitary where it is then secreted when necessary to the kidneys. This then affects the osmotic pressure in the extracelluar fluids. The despatched antidiuretic hormone in the kidneys will then act to either promote or demote the need for water retention with the subsequent lower or higher osmotic pressure. Thankfully, it all works automatically. For the average person, in temperate weather conditions, partaking in moderate activity will have a daily water (food or drink) requirement of 2.5 litres.

The body water supply '**In**' comes from:

- food: fruits and vegetables have a very high percentage of water, whereas butters, oils, chocolate, cookies and cakes much lower water contents
- fluids: water being the only true drink, all others can be classed as either foods (milk, fruit juices etc.) or stimulants (tea, coffee, alcohol)
- the body's internal metabolism

The body water supply '**Out**' goes from:

- products of the body waste disposal processes
- through skin perspiration, temperature regulation
- in the air you breathe out

Water Balance
Therefore, for a person consuming balanced meals, they require just over **one** litre of water to keep the body water balance stable:

In

Fluids	4 small glasses* of water (= **one** litre)
Food	5
Metabolism	1
Total	**10**

*1 glass = 250ml

Out

Waste matter	5 and a half glasses
Skin	3
Lungs	1 and a half
Total	**10**

Find out more about water balancing in Chapter 6 – The fountain of youth, there you will discover the enormous importance to your physical, emotional, and psychological health of water balancing, the factors which affect it, and how you can find solutions that will greatly enhance your health.

Nature's way
Earth, once upon a time billions of years ago, had an atmosphere of feverishly hot and vibrant gases. The eventual cooling of Earth and the subsequent coming together of hydrogen and oxygen was the birth of water (in the shape of steam to start with). A further cooling of the Earth, gave rise to rock formations, and after the steam had condensed into rain, a place for the water (this time in liquid form) to settle.

> It is believed that when the first rains fell upon Earth
> they lasted for hundreds of years.
>
> *Health-Warrior*

Moreover, after millions of years later, a few more rock formations and larger amounts of water, there was a clearly defined land and sea mass, similar to the world today. The seas, lakes, rivers and their likes, cover the Earth with nearly 75% water. Water vapour has been around for millions of years filling the air and clouds, and overseeing the first forms of life. Remarkably, even after all this time it has not been used up and the water cycle continues to provide all living things with life. Therefore, it is very possible that a mouthful of water consumed by dinosaurs millions of years ago could find its way into the water supply you use today.

Without the water cycle, namely the resultant actions of the sun, air, water, and gravitational forces, this Earth would be uninhabitable just as other planets in Earth's solar system are. The water cycle provides the means for the movement of water from Earth into the atmosphere, and back down to Earth again. There is always a large amount of water vapour to be found in the atmosphere awaiting the ride back to Earth. The oceans make up 97% of the Earths water supply with the remaining 3% freshwater. Of this 3% over three quarters is found in ice and the glaciers; 20% in ground water; with only 1% being easy-access surface water. Lakes represent half of the easy-access freshwater to be found, with the rest being shared between: soil 38%, atmosphere 8%, rivers 1%, and within living beings 1%. Water in its 'purest' form is never found in nature and has to be produced by way of a distillation processes in laboratories, because minerals (which the body requires for optimum living) use it as a home and transport system. This positive capacity of water to act as an excellent 'home' for minerals is abused by pollutants who attach to it, to become a source of human illness, disease, and death.

Amber nectar of the Gods

Ever since humans realised the importance of water to their existence, it has represented a special place in their beliefs, religions, myths, and fairy tales. From Egypt to India, and the Americas to Australasia, the sacred writings of the Qur'an, Bible, and Torah, to the earliest found human etchings and pyramid texts; water has been regarded as very powerful. Water was seen as, among other things, Holy water, life giving, a symbol of regeneration, a pagan of worship, a cleanser of sins, and as reason for sacrificial rites.

> The *Physiologus* states that when the eagle has grown old and its eyes have become dim and darkened, it flies upward towards the sun until it has scorched its wings and purged away the film from its eyes; then it descends to the earth and plunges three times into a spring of pure water. Thus it recovers its sight and renews its youth.
>
> *Physiologus was compiled by an*
> *Alexandrian Greek*

In Indian Sanskrit texts water was believed to be a drink of immortality. The Egyptian tablets of Aeth wrote that 'souls are weighed in silence, as gold and silver are weighed in pure water'. Other pyramid texts indicated that the Egyptians believed water to be magical, 'the water I give to you is the water of eternal youth'. Millions of Hindus revere the 'Mother' Ganges as the 'life-giving river', not only because it provides food but because it is a sacred place where you can wash away sins and find eternal peace on its banks in death.

The dark side of water
Throughout the ages, and in recent times, global tragedies have shown how lethal water can be. A tsunami can wipe out towns and villages in seconds; floods can take lives and belongings in their path; hurricane storms leave devastation in their wake; a drought can reshape populations. Added to this, is the everyday damage caused by normal rainfall, snow, and hail, and the fact that it can also carry diseases such as typhoid, dysentery, and cholera, and you are presented with a picture of damage which costs trillions and more importantly, hundreds of thousands of deaths, injuries, and human suffering.

Chapter 5

Liquidity

From the ancient civilisations to modern cities, water has determined where people choose to live. Ancient nomads would pitch their tents from oasis to oasis and still do to this day. As populations rose so did, the ways of transporting water from its source to people, and lands flourished. Egyptians used open canals to transport the water closer to arable lands and homes; the ancient Greeks and Romans used variations of the aqueduct system; and in 1582 London, England, the first reservoir and pump systems were introduced.

> ...consider the qualities of the waters, for as they differ from one another in taste and weight, so also do they differ much in their qualities...for water contributes much towards health.
>
> *On Airs, Waters, and Places*
> *Hippocrates*

Water was essential in choosing where food was produced, as the Earth only has 7% of arable lands available for food production. Industry utilises water to produce electricity and power for homes and factories; and most of all global transportation could not take place without utilising water.

> An oil giants needs close to forty litres of water to refine just four litres of petrol.
>
> *Health-Warrior*

Use and supply

The average person will consume on average 400 litres of water per day living in the city. This can include anything from drinking it, house cleaning, cooking, gardening, and personal cleanliness; a quota has also been allocated to indirect uses like watering and cleaning of communal areas, and emergency services. The usage amounts vary enormously from person to person, neighbourhood to neighbourhood, and country to country. The disparity revolves around the differences of environment and socioeconomic factors. For example, developed and developing countries have an alarmingly high thirst for, and usage of water. The average American will consume on average 570 litres per day. More than 450 billion litres (and rising) of water is consumed by the Americans alone. Moreover, not having a local supply of water is no longer a major obstacle, as San Diego, in the state of Los Angeles, United States, has its water transported via a 242-mile aqueduct from the Colorado River.

The global water use is steadily rising as populations continue to expand, and billions of litres of water are temporarily lost from the water cycle, and cannot be immediately reused.

Water conservation

Water is replenishable, as the water cycle has proved for millions of years. The problems start to occur when primary sources are contaminated or when the recycled water is of an inferior quality.

There are many parts of the globe now where the sprawling cities are creating situations where the supply of water cannot fulfil the demands being placed on it; with many cities suffering water shortages and are forced to put in place contingency plans to conserve water such as hosepipe bans or temporary total stoppages of supply. The responsibility of those who use water (that is everybody) is to actively conserve water and avoid polluting or contaminating it. You need to find ways to achieve a more efficient usage of water and here are a few ideas to get you started (if you are not doing so already):

- Vegetables and fruit should be washed in a bowl and not under a running tap
- Reuse the leftover water for other tasks such as watering house plants and flushing the toilet
- Use the minimum amount of water required when you boil water in saucepans and kettles; that way, you'll save energy as well as water
- If you have to, only use washing machines and dishwashers when they are full. ('half-load' or 'economy' use more than half the water and electricity of the full load).
- Do not leave the tap running while you brush your teeth, shave or wash your hands, as this can waste up to five litres of water per minute

- When showering, turn the water off in between the foaming, scrubbing, and rinsing stages. A five-minute shower uses about a third of the water of a bath. But remember that power showers can use more water than a bath in less than five minutes
- Use 'low flush' toilets for lower water usage. For older toilets modify it, to use less (as 40% of all household usage is from the toilet)
- Put waste materials such as, cotton wool or tissues in a waste bin rather than flushing them down the toilet
- Keep your plumbing well maintained, as dripping taps can waste up to four litres of water a day
- Insulate pipes for both energy saving and to avoid cracks and leaks in cold months
- Reduce the use of garden sprinklers and hoses for watering
- Utilise rainwater; as much rainfall as possible should be collected for reuse (e.g. roof guttering and piping should lead to water storage containers)
- Wash the car yourself with a bucket and sponge, and not waste litres of water at the carwash

Polluted water is dead water

In the year 1700, the average person in Europe could expect only two litres of water per day, and in those miserly two litres, they had to try to avoid the diseases typhoid, dysentery, and cholera. Today, water pollution, the process of making water or soil dangerously dirty and not suitable for people to use, is still an ever-present danger but in a different guises; for example, it is estimated that 100 million people worldwide are drinking water that contains substantial amounts of sewage effluent.

Water pollution has many sources, such as inadequately treated sewage, fertilisers, silt, organic matter, petroleum, radioactive waste, heat, waste materials (such as metals, plastics, solvents, dyes, and inks), pathogens (microscopic waterborne chemicals), and pesticides. When you acknowledge the 'pollution footprint' that each person leaves on the environment, then you can truly appreciate the scale of the problem at hand; for example, each American citizen will add more than a ton of new hazardous waste to the environment each year, making them the highest per capita waste producers in the world.

What is polluting your water?

"Water, water everywhere, but not a drop to drink"
from the Rhyme of the Ancient Mariner

Both domestic and industrial sewage and fertilisers contain nutrients such as nitrates and phosphates, and as any keen gardener will know, these nutrients will stimulate growth in plants and flowers. However, when these nutrients find their way into streams, ponds, and waterways they can cause damage to the ecosystem by over stimulating growth in the plants and algae. This in turn, will produce a lack of oxygenated water for the expanding ecosystem and can result in the eventual death of aquatic life, due to this artificial clogging of streams, ponds, and waterways.

While another danger to aquatic life, comes in the shape of excessive silt and soils from agriculture, construction sites, factories, and eroding rivers and rains. These pollution sources cause an unnatural shifting of natural ecosystems, and the sediment produced will inhibit the respiration of fish, the growth of plants, and alter the physical depths of the waterways. The 'dirty' water also diminishes the amount of sunlight that can penetrate the water, the absence of which can inhibit the growth of the aquatic plants that normally furnish the water with oxygen.

Organic matter (such as animal sewage and feed, leaves, and garden refuse) will again undergo breakdown in the water and reduce the oxygen supplies in it. In the United States alone, 22% of water supplies have been found to contain at least one volatile organic substance.

Oil is spilt on a minute scale every time a ship transports it; though the amount may be insignificant, the fact that no oil spill can ever be 100% eliminated from the water, adds a greater significance to this fact. Oil spills devastate environments and require a further introduction of 'new' chemicals to the polluted environment for the 'clean-up' purposes.

Radioactivity has always been part of the natural environment. The dangers, however, start to occur when humans try to harness radioactivity for their inexhaustible energy requirements, and from the industrial, medical, and scientific use of radioactive materials. The radioactive substances produced from the waste materials will leave behind a legacy of dangerous pollution for the future generations, and are extremely destructive to human health and environment for those living presently. On April 26, 1986, the Chernobyl nuclear power plant in the old Soviet Union was the centre of a nuclear disaster. Full details of which may never be disclosed but a meltdown at the plant occurred and exposed radioactive materials. Cancer, birth defects, skin, and respiratory diseases are to name only a few of the dangers of radioactivity exposure. Though many scientists predict there to be many other illnesses and diseases attributed to the accident, as the medical effects of radioactive exposure take years to become apparent. With a shelf life of thousands of years, radioactive wastes pose a greater immediate problem. The safe disposal of these wastes has so far proved elusive to science, and created a dangerous and expensive problem to industry.

When you switch on any electrical appliance the energy you use will be produced at an electric power plant in your vicinity. The rising energy needs of people has created an increasing threat from the heat produced by the electric power plants as they burn fossil fuels or nuclear fuel to provide this energy. As this process releases a considerable amount of heat, the power plant will usually locate itself near a supply of water, which the power plants use for heat-dissipation purposes. The heat is a pollutant because increased water temperature results in the deaths of many aquatic organisms.

Relatively new on the scene and possibly the most destructive pollutants, are the microscopic waterborne chemicals. It is an environmental time bomb waiting to happen for the people of the 21st century. In Milwaukee, United States, a waterborne chemical incident in 1993 caused 403,000 reported illnesses and fifty-four deaths. Pathogens are one such type of pollutant. They travel in the guise of bacteria and viruses, with the ability to cause wide-ranging illnesses from typhoid to respiratory diseases. They enter through untreated sewage, storm drains, septic tanks, farm waste, and dumped sewage from ships and boats.

The United States reports over nine million cases of waterborne diseases per year.

Industry in its attempt for increased efficiency, in order to keep up with an expanding population and subsequent increasing demand, has much to answer for. Like the dumping of oils, toxic chemicals, and other harmful industrial wastes; mining and oil-drilling operations, corrosive acid wastes; agricultural fertilisers, insecticides, and pesticides. The agricultural pesticides are designed to protect crops from insects, weeds, fungi, and some animals. The pesticide can withstand rain and therefore can inhabit the environment for a much longer period then is actually required. Another problem arises when pests develop genetic resistance to the pesticides used, causing an increase in the quantity used, and an increase in the variations of the pesticides available to the farmer. It would take fifteen years to clear Africa of all the agricultural chemicals with recognised harmful hazards. There is a wide variation of government policy towards pesticides, with a certain pesticide having been banned in the United States and most other countries, while it continues to be manufactured and used in other parts of the world.

Dioxins are environmental 'serial pollutants', they are very dangerous and have an adept ability to extend there stay either in humans or the environment. Once in humans they dissolve their way into fat and have a half-life of seven years. There are some thirty known dioxin compounds which are significantly toxic and are found in among others, soil, water, and sediment. (They are also found in foods and you shall meet these serial pollutants' again in Part three – Nourishment). These compounds are by-products of many industrial processes including paper manufacturing, and some pesticides. The biggest contributor of dioxins into the environment is the waste incinerators.

> One particular dioxin, 'Agent Orange' was extensively
> used during the Vietnam War.

Health hazards of the dioxins to humans are many and one of the most serious is cancer; but it can also affect the immune system, central nervous system, and reproductive functions. With these kinds of hazards, it is surprising that there are only twenty laboratories in the world with the technology to measure dioxins in human blood.

The World Health Organisation (WHO) publishes guideline values for chemicals that are of health significance in drinking water, and these range from Acrylamide to Xylenes. Dr Lee Jong-Wook, a Director General of the WHO has stated that 'Water and sanitation is one of the primary drivers of public health. I often refer to it as "Health 101", which means that once we can secure access to clean water and to adequate sanitation facilities for all people, irrespective of the difference in their living conditions, a huge battle against all kinds of diseases will be won.'

However, until then the cases of illnesses, diseases, and deaths continue to be documented unabated. The simple fact is that, only 10% of pesticides have been tested by toxicologists and have a complete file of information on their health hazards. A third of the pesticides available have not been tested for toxicity at all. The problem is even greater with commercially used chemicals where 80% have never been tested and little or nothing is known about their health hazards.

> There are one million new chemicals introduced into the
> world each year, and everyday 4,000 new potential
> hazards to contend with. Everyday people are dying with
> a cocktail of chemicals in their blood.

Arsenic in water has well documented adverse health effects and in the WHO report on the issue, identified cancer (skin, lung, bladder, and kidney), vomiting, abdominal pains, and diarrhoea attributable to arsenic contaminated water. China, India, and Bangladesh have problems with arsenic in their drinking water. Bangladesh alone, had suffered up to 270,000 deaths from cancer attributed to such polluted water in 2001. However, it is not just restricted to developing or under-developed countries, as it is reported that in the United States that up to thirteen million people are exposed to arsenic contaminated water.

The United Kingdom has had its fair share of water related incidents, with one of the more significant ones occurring in Camelford. In July 1988, twenty tonnes of aluminium sulphate, a neurotoxin, was mistakenly tipped into a reservoir of 'ready for public use' water. The polluted water was then released to 20,000 people in the Camelford area. In an investigation, which tracked the events and effects of the incident, found that the neurotoxin caused brain damage, with symptoms to that specific area such as memory loss, reduced concentration, and lower IQ levels.

In his revealing new book Autism, Brain and Environment, the scientist Richard Lathe examines the link between the rapid rises over the last two decades in autism and the increased levels of pollution. Lathe attributes some of the autism cases to an increase in environmental toxins: pesticides, PCBs (from plastics), and particularly heavy metals including mercury and lead (both known neurotoxins).

Bottled water – Is it really a safe haven?
Those of you who have read about and listened to the long running problems regarding clean water supply and are not too concerned because you predominantly drink only bottled water, thinking that it is a 'safer' option, then you may need to revisit the water problem once again. The 1989 United Kingdom Water Act requires that tap water is tested at every treatment stage. It is tested daily and against fifty-seven parameters, which can detect up to ninety different chemical substances, with the records of the tests available to the public.

Americans consume over fifteen billion litres of bottled water each year.

Are bottled waters as clean? Bottled waters are split in law into two types: 'Mineral' and 'Spring' waters. The Natural Mineral Waters Association claims the parameters call for mineral waters to be tested for only thirteen chemicals and bacteria - less than one quarter as many substances as are tested for in tap water. There are also no requirements that mineral water be tested daily or even weekly and the test results, when they happen, of the mineral waters are not available to the public. 'Spring' water has no specific legislation, and therefore, there are water bottles on shelves today that have had no analysis at all.

The World Health Organisation issued a warning regarding bottled water as it found contamination on many levels. Some bottled water contained traces of lead and arsenic, others bacteria, virus, and parasites; even identified physical objects such as glass and metal. In addition, in a similar study in Cleveland, Ohio, a well-respected medical journal found that sampled bottled water contained ten-times more bacteria when compared with ordinary tap water. The size of a company should not be taken as a mark of quality assurance either, as Coca-Cola a global brand with a multi-million dollar turnover, in 2004 introduced bottled water to the market under the name Dasani. The bottles were sold to the unsuspecting public as 'pure' water. As the first bottles were being consumed, every bottle in circulation was recalled at great expense, because the so-called 'pure' water was tap water, and more seriously, contained a cancer causing chemical called bromate, which was registered at twice the legal limit.

In a recent report by the Food Commission, it found that some samples of bottled water had travelled 10,000 miles (16,000 km) before reaching United Kingdom supermarket consumers. Europe in general, is suffering from water shortages and safety issues, and has done so for many years. It is currently the 'number one' factor in tackling health problems across many European countries. Nitrogen pollution, for example, is a growing problem as farmers try to etch out more produce from fertiliser-saturated lands. Over the past decade, all cooperating European countries have reported water related diseases.

One billion people are without access to clean drinking water and a further 2.6 billion without adequate sanitation. The large numbers result in 5 million deaths every year from the lack of safe drinking water. The illnesses and diseases include diarrhoea (1.8 million deaths per year), malaria (396 million episodes per year), hepatitis A (1.5 million cases), and in China alone 26 million people are affected by fluorsis. The situation is only likely to be inflated by the growing population, rapid urbanisation (as countries like China continue to expand at alarming rates), pollution, inefficient water supplies (leaks, illegal tapping), industry demands, and wastage.

What is next on the horizon?
Pharmaceuticals companies currently dispose of their waste materials in random and unsafe ways; and they been shown to end up in local wastewater treatment plants. University of Buffalo chemists testing wastewater in the Western New York (United States) areas identified for the first time the metabolites of two antibiotics (sulfamethoxazole and trimethoprim, commonly prescribed antibiotics) in this water. Also identified was a synthetic estrogen, a common ingredient in birth control pills and in hormone replacement therapy. The concern is that the chemical compounds could end up in tap water with potential adverse effects to humans and the environment. With water contaminated by antibiotics and their metabolites, you could be facing a population with an increased antibiotic resistance, a confused internal system (as their

body functions are affected by the synthetic hormones), and water treatment system that is not designed to cope with this new pollutant.

> ...treatment facilities don't monitor or measure organic micro contaminants like residues of pharmaceuticals and active ingredients of personal care product...The pharmaceuticals we monitored are not degraded completely in the treatment plants; most of them are just transformed into other compounds that still may have adverse eco toxicological effects.
>
> *Diana Aga, Ph.D.*
> *University of Buffalo's College of Arts and Sciences*

What can you do to stop water pollution?
If you start making small positive contributions in your own life, it will add to the worldwide collective fight against water pollution and its many dangerous and life-threatening illnesses and diseases. It is every human beings right to have access to clean water. Rainwater will collect and carry many pollutants such as sediment, pet waste, pesticides, fertilizers, motor vehicle products (such as oil and grease), and garden waste, from roofs, paved surfaces, and soils.

Here are things you can do today to reduce water pollution:

- Reduce the usage of motor vehicles
- If you have to use a car then, keep it to one per household
- Keep the vehicles well maintained to avoid leaks of substances such as oil, grease, and fuel
- Wash your car with less cleaning products, and use buckets (not the hose) for the water
- Clean up after your pets
- Reduce the use of toxic chemicals for 'house cleaning'
- Use environmentally friendly DIY paints, varnishes, and solvents, and dispose of them as per label instructions
- Avoid disposing of medicines, creams, lotions and potions via the water supply
- Recycle, renew, repair, before sending anything to the refuse incinerator
- Recycle all garden waste, including grass and tree cuttings, hence, reinvesting your time, water, and nutrients, back into your garden
- Direct rainwater to collecting areas for later use
- Reduce use of pesticides, fertilizers, and watering

- Choose plants and trees that are native and well adapted to your area (for example, do not maintain a lavish lawn or exotic plants unless rain water can sustain them)
- Use organic products
- Avoid introducing large areas of paved areas into your garden; a natural habitat is more beautiful and Earth friendly

Enter the stimulants

Stimulants can be viewed as being polluted or contaminated water. In almost all cases, the stimulants will disrupt your water supply and subsequently your optimum hydration and more worryingly, interfere with your normal brain functions.

In normal conditions the two most vital areas of your body, the brain and central nervous system make use of neurotransmitters by sending and receiving messages to affect feeling; the process is a balanced one. In the case of stimulants and drugs, the neurotransmitters reacting to the presence of the stimulant compounds, send too many messages into your system than you can cope with. You in turn, experience the initial 'high' or 'energy buzz'. In the meantime, your body actively strives to return to a balanced state, trying to limit the 'high' feelings. This is one of the reasons, why in time you will need more quantities of the same stimulant to get a similar effect. This is why; subsequent cups of coffee will never have the same effect as the initial ones do, or did.

This is the same for any stimulant such as caffeine, nicotine, alcohol, and cocaine or any other narcotic. What happens is that any period of over stimulation (too many messages released into your system), results with the body fighting back to regain its balance by closing down some of the receptors for the messages sent. You do not get the message, and do not get the 'high' as desired, and therefore, crave greater quantities of the stimulant to get a similar effect. Moreover, the more you have of the stimulant the more your body closes down the receptors until you no longer get any 'high' feelings from the stimulant at all; to the point that you require a 'fix' just to feel normal and forget those desires to feel good.

Addiction is at the end of this downward spiralling road, and once you realise there is no good for you there, you try to quit using the stimulant or drug. To begin with, you will feel low because you have upset the balance of the neurotransmitters; and without the stimulant or drug there are no 'good' feeling messages being sent. This is the withdrawal suffered in any addiction recovery. However, as mentioned before, the body seeks balance and the withdrawal period is anywhere between, a number of days for caffeine to weeks for nicotine, before the neurotransmitters are back to normal and have similar amounts of sending and receiving messages.

What is the chemical 1, 3, 7 – trimethylxanthine more commonly known as? It is known as caffeine; it is a substance that exists naturally in coffee beans, tealeaves, cocoa (chocolate products), and cola nuts. It can be produced synthetically subsequently being used consumer products such as soft drinks, energy supplements, and pharmaceutical products such as cold remedies, diuretics, pain remedies, stimulants, and weight control. It is a central nervous system stimulant and a diuretic.

> There is no nutritional requirement of the body for the chemical caffeine.
>
> *Health-Warrior*

The upside of caffeine is that, within minutes, you will experience increased energy, a heightened mental and physical ability, and possibly a better mood. The considerable downside means you may have the urge to go to the toilet within the hour (it is a diuretic after all), and start to feel drowsy, irritable, and have the desire for another 'fix' within the next two. These are some of the effects of caffeine usage in both the short and long terms (sometimes referred to as 'caffeine intoxication'):

- restlessness
- insomnia
- headaches
- nervous irritability / agitation
- digestion problems
- increases in heart rate
- increases in blood pressure
- dehydration
- adrenal gland problems
- addiction
- withdrawal symptoms
- toxic poisons from pesticides used in growing the plants

What is your caffeine fix?
Coffee is the number one caffeine fiend and in the United States alone, consumption equates to two daily cups of espresso for every man, woman, or child. An unimaginable, fourteen million kilograms of coffee per year are playing havoc with your body balance! A Starbucks Grande has a massive 550mg of caffeine, instant coffee up to 108 mg, and an espresso 100 mg.

Decaffeinated products are not the answer either, as they harbour other stimulants such as theophylline and threobromine, and you could be exposed to the other harsh chemicals used in the decaffeinating process. Teas have all the same caffeine downsides and contain tannin, which can hamper absorption of vitamins and minerals. A three minute brewed tea has up to 46 mg of caffeine; and Ice tea has 36mg.

> Fizzy drinks make you fat: one fizzy drink per day
> would result in a weight gain of over six kilograms in
> one year!

Fizzy drinks hit you with both caffeine and sugar. Excess sugar has the same 'energy buzz' and any other stimulant and if over used similar negative downsides. In addition, chemicals like aspartame, a common additive in colas, cause toxic stimulation to the brain. Here are a few caffeine amounts of selected soft drinks: Coca-cola diet coke has 46 mg of caffeine; Dr Pepper 40mg; Dr Pepper sugar-free 40mg; Pepsi 38mg; Diet Pepsi 36mg. In May 2006, the global company, Coca-Cola signed a 'voluntary' agreement to remove all its fizzy drinks from elementary and middle schools in the United States, under pressure from concerns about the fizzy drinks effects on children's health; for some countries however, the soft drink giant is still an immovable caffeine and sugar-fix at a arms distance from the classroom.

Energy drinks, relative new comers to the caffeine scene, have seen massive popularity, and introduced a new global brand in the process, Red Bull. In the UK alone, it is a £1 billion market, having grabbed a 20% share of the soft drinks market. The caffeine contents vary between companies but the Red Bull energy drink contains 90mg of caffeine per small can.

Chocolate has the treble hit of caffeine, sugar, and saturated and trans fats, and all their downsides respectively. In addition, can carry residues of pesticides used in their growing. Baking chocolate has 35mg of caffeine, while sweet or dark chocolate has 20mg.

> 90% of the UK drinks alcohol and the bill comes to £40
> billion.

Alcohol is an addictive 'drug-stimulant' with initial reactions of pleasure and a lowering of inhibitions. The 'good' feeling neurotransmitters are at work again by first releasing the messages of happiness, then the feelings of relaxation. Secondary reactions include irritability to hostility, and depressive moods. Within twenty-four hours feelings of nausea, headaches, gastrointestinal problems, and dehydration, can be suffered; also know as the hangover.

> Dehydration can reduce important body functions such
> as, sexual activity.

Alcohol has been linked as a direct or indirect cause to many illnesses, diseases, and deaths. Below are a few of those alcohol derived health issues:

- Increased risk of cancer
- Blood pressure changes
- Increased insulin secretion
- Higher glucose disposal
- Hyperglycaemia
- Reduced bone density (cause of osteoporosis)
- Increased toxicity
- Accelerating of aging process
- Reduction of brain functions
- Depression
- Addiction

Chapter 6

The fountain of youth

'Clean' water is your simple key to open doors to deep and wondrous treasures. Behind each door, there are treasures of rejuvenation, regeneration, an inner strength and resistance, a fluidity of thought and action, and a perpetual force of wellness. Once you've secured the treasures of clean water, you will carry a natural, radiating glow that people cannot walk past without noticing, and have the feeling of, for want of a less clichéd phrase, the ability to walk (in health and well-being terms) on water.

> Every human has the responsibility, individually and collectively, to reclaim the right to have a direct supply of clean, pollution-free water.
>
> *Health-Warrior*

The water balance revisited
This is where it all takes place. Your water balance is the foundation to great health. Take care of this and your body will take care of you. Water is the only drink, which quenches thirst (all others are foods or stimulants). High water content foods provide excellent water supply, as most are greater than 70% water-rich, and house the essential nutrients for the body. As seen previously, an average inactive 70kg person eating a well balanced diet will have a water requirement of 2.5 litres, of which four glasses (250ml) would be drinking water and five portions of fruit and/or vegetables. As one becomes more active, the water requirement also increases. (The benefits of physical activity are enormous and are resoundingly endorsed by the Health-Warrior and will be looked at in detail in Part five – Made for motion).

Thirst things first
Thirst is, under normal conditions, a very reliable indicator of water requirements. The problems start to occur when people cannot decipher

between the signals of thirst and hunger, which originate from the brain structure, the hypothalamus. The hypothalamus is directly concerned with among other things, a person's feeding (hunger, satiety) and drinking (water intake, thirst, and salt balance) behaviours. It is especially tuned to receiving signals from the body senses: smell, taste, and vision; and will act in order to maintain homeostasis (the body's balanced state). For most, the thirst sensation is felt in the mouth, as the saliva starts to become more viscous in its properties (and a prolonged headache or such like effects will occur if ignored). A healthy water supply is a regular one, and one where supply swings such as floods or droughts are not common occurrences.

> For a person undertaking a prolonged bout of activity and undergoing heavy water and mineral losses through sweating, thirst ceases to be a reliable indicator for the body water requirements. As the 'thirst' feeling will kick in too late and will not account for the extra minerals lost in the activity.

Drink your water at room temperature, in small mouthfuls allowing time for the water to saturate all areas inside of your mouth. Hot or cold-water temperatures only have an irritating effect on the body, as it tries to get the water back to a more manageable temperature for use.

> You are either 'drinking' for liquid replacement or 'eating' for nutrient replacement; you should avoid mixing the two.
>
> *Health-Warrior*

The ideal times for water intake are in between meals. However, in most cultures there seems to be an ingrained tradition, which suggests there is the need to drink some kind of liquid refreshment either, immediately before, during, or after eating. Consuming liquids at mealtimes only succeeds in interfering with the first stage of digestion that takes place in the mouth, while also giving you the ability to wash down dry (water and nutrient deficient) foods such as butters, oils, chocolate, breads, pastries, cookies, cakes, and biscuits you should be otherwise moderating. This interference in the first stage of digestion will wash away the usefulness of the saliva in your mouth. The saliva in your mouth is an active part of the first stage of digestion, and if allowed to, performs with stealth effectiveness. Lubricating food is its obvious function, but there are other important ones to note, as saliva will

- dissolve the food particles, in order for the taste receptors to receive the 'taste sensation'; The taste receptors will only respond to dissolved food, so washing your food down or swallowing it without chewing it will render the food tasteless. And more worrying is the fact that if the taste buds do not receive these messages then it could delay the feeling of satiety and consequently, you will not feel 'full' and are more likely to eat more

- use its digestive enzyme to start to break down carbohydrates in the mouth which enhances your taste sensations
- help to protect your teeth and gums with its anti-bacterial enzyme

A good watering

Here is an example of an ordinary day of water intake for a 30-year-old male, weighing 70kg, in average weather conditions who is moderately active, and follows a well-balanced diet. The food intake assumes no excesses of minerals such as salt, or the consumption of alcohol or stimulants. The ideal water intake would be four glasses of water or one litre, and look like this:

On waking	1 average glasses (250ml) of water
Mid Morning	1 glass of water
Late afternoon	1 glass of water
Evening	1 glass of water

Many factors can change your water requirements such as your lifestyle activity levels or diet, your environment such as climate and temperature, and your physical characteristics such as age, gender, and body composition. In general, the younger you are the higher your metabolic rate and the more water your body will require. Women (especially during pregnancy) will require more water than their male counterpart, whereas older adults will tend to consume less water as they get older.

Here are a few expert tips on how to maximise your water benefits for optimum health

- Your first glass of water should be drunk the moment you wake up – hydrating and cleansing your system
- Sip mouthful of water at room temperatures
- Avoid the very hot and cold drinks as they are just irritating to the body
- Take care to not drink at mealtimes
- Excessive salt should be avoided
- Avoid stimulants

- Avoid excessive water or liquids in the evening (otherwise, sleep will be disturbed)
- For increased activity, increase both water and high water content foods

The table below gives you an idea of the amount of water you should aim to drink (assuming average weather conditions, no use of diuretics such as tea or coffee), partake in moderate physical activity, and no hydration related illnesses or diseases:

Calories per day (kcal)	Water quantity (litres)	High water content food (portion)
2000	1	5
2250	1.25	6
2500	1.5	7
2750	1.75	8
3000	2	9

Note: For higher calorie consumptions seek the advice of a qualified nutritionist

Water, physical activity, and exercise
Not only do you have to replace the water lost during physical activity or exercise but you also have to replace the minerals in the plasma concentration. A moderate physical activity session lasting over an hour will lose between 0.5 to 1.0 litres of water (perspiration). To restore body balance, you must drink between 25 to 50% greater supplies of water and replace the mineral plasma concentration lost, to avoid dehydration. Drinking only plain water will dilute the mineral plasma concentration in your body and simply cause you to urinate more and not rehydrate your body. To overcome this, consume an isotonic drink, which will replace both the water and mineral content of the perspiration lost through the moderate physical activity.

> Make your own isotonic drink; for a one-litre bottle: mix one part fruit juice with three parts water, and add half a teaspoon of salt; give in a shake and that is all there is to it.
>
> *Health-Warrior*

Older and wiser
Aging is partly a dehydrating process; and if you want to delay this process then you will need to use water to unlock the secrets of your youthfulness. Your ability to keep your body adequately hydrated, as you get older, will help you to look younger for your age, have plenty of

energy, and give you the platform to fight off illness and disease more effectively.

> Ageing, for instance, is a dehydrating process: as you age the water content in your body and brain decreases. So drinking enough water can slow down the ageing process.
>
> *Patrick Holford & Dr Hyla Cass*
> *Natural Highs*

The problem is there are a few physiological barriers you will need to overcome first before you can adequately hydrate your body. As you age your internal controls among other things, will gradually decrease your metabolic rate (the rate at which your body expends energy from your food at rest), reduce the thirst sensations you experience, effect your ability to control your internal body temperatures (you will not sweat as much), and reduce the working capacity of your kidneys. The slowing of your metabolic rate will also reduce the ability to renew body tissue and the ability to eliminate toxic waste efficiently. So it will not be a simple process of the more water you drink, the more you will be hydrated and the greater the delay to the aging process, because these physiological changes to your body will need to be addressed before you can enjoy the youthful benefits of more water.

A first and highly beneficial step will be to maintain and try to increase your metabolic rate by making changes in your nourishment and by introducing the right types of physical activity. Your nourishment should include foods, which will energise your body and pack it with age-fighting nutrients, while the right type of physical activity will increase your muscle mass, strength, and reduce fat gain. For the bigger picture however, you need to be aware that aging is a complex process and no one action will provide you with all the transformations you desire. This book covers the most important components (a person's genetics aside) of the aging process, breathing, hydration, nourishment, sleep, and activity. The key to reversing the aging process is to look at all these components as one, as acting on one and not the other, will not provide the exponential benefits on offer, if you were to act on all of them.

Part three

Nourishment

By far the largest part of this book is devoted to the practice of nourishment and with good reason, as it is also the one area, which has been, and continues to be the one most tampered with. As we have previously stated, the human body has remained relatively unchanged for the last few tens of thousands of years but what we eat has become virtually unrecognisable to that what was being eaten as near as a few decades ago. Coincidently, during this same period, a host of diseases have been introduced into modern life because of these nutritional changes.

Poor nutritional habits can expose a person to bouts of fatigue, irritability, cravings, mood swings, lapses in memory and concentration, headaches, difficulties in sleeping lacking motivation, and suffer issues such as food allergies, sensitivities, skin ailments, bad breath, faulty digestion, water retention, appetite disruptions, and dental problems. Furthermore, the longer-term effects of poor nutritional habits have been associated with major 'modern' diseases such as coronary heart disease, diabetes, cancer, high blood pressure, and the more obvious one, obesity.

After air and water, how your body is nourished is the next vital element to, firstly your survival and secondly, your physical and mental good health and well-being. Your body is made up of trillions of cells, which are the fundamental elements of life. They operate on the nutrients you supply and this allows them to function efficiently, repairing, growing, communicating, and responding where required to the signals from the body senses and the environment. By understanding how food and nutrients affect the health of your cells, you not only know which foods are beneficial, but how and why a food plan that features nutrient-rich whole foods free of toxic chemicals and additives, can positively transform your health. Food, which has been processed and removed beyond its natural state (such as the use of additives, genetic modification, pollution, antibiotics, and improper storage or cooking), can be viewed as tampered or doctored food. This 'unreal' food is riding on a massive tide of high sugar, high fat (saturated and trans fatty acids), and high salt which is a force against your desires for good health and well-being. This force is manipulating your food, making it addictive and devoid of nutrients, creating an environment encouraging excessive eating.

This goes some way to explain why food trends and consumer behaviour continues to move towards unhealthy foods despite the overwhelming evidence of damage they can cause to health. Why else would someone consciously choose to eat foods that will eventually reduce their quality of living and ultimately shorten their life?

In the previous chapters, you have discovered how small changes in your interactions with air and water can lead to positive change in your life; your nourishment is no different. It is the collective power of these small changes, which will introduce you to an energised, youthful, and disease-free lifestyle. The following chapters will reveal, among other things, how to identify your food requirements for optimum health. Introducing you to the nutrient packed MaxLife foods with healing, energising, and de-aging properties, which help you to pinpoint the dangers that lurk in food and provide practical tips in how to avoid them, and empower you to lead the fight against the forces of ill health and disease.

Chapter 7

Bite-size basics

Energy is essential to sustain your body, and nutrition is the source of this energy. It is the base from, which your biological and chemical reactions are initiated, and also the body's repairing and renewing functions use this food energy to do their work. The food you eat is broken down to its smallest elements and these chemical reactions release the energy, which sustains body functions, such as respiration, brain signals, circulation, and physical activity. One of the by-products of these chemical reactions is heat; this in turn helps with maintenance of your body thermoregulation.

In simple terms your energy balance expenditure is:

Energy balance   =   energy intake   −   energy expenditure

At the most basic level, if your energy intake (nutrition) is greater than your energy expenditure (metabolism, body functions, and physical activity) then you will have a positive energy balance, and you will be liable to put on weight mostly in the shape of fat. Conversely, if your energy intake is less than your expenditure, you will have a negative energy balance. Depending on the size of the negative balance, you will either maintain your body weight or lose some of it. This simple equation determines the changes in your body weight, and holds the key to sustained health and longevity.

The energy bank

All the foods eaten will be broken down in to smaller elements, into 'currency', which the body can use. Once the digestive system is presented with the correct currency, it will accept the currency transfer and deposit it into the blood stream to be transported and used immediately or saved for another day. This currency is the fuel a body need to operate and it can be measured in terms of kilocalories (kcal) or simply called calories.

Currency converter

One gram of	Calories (kcal)
Fat	9
Protein	4
Carbohydrate	4
Alcohol	7

Your body needs a minimum amount of currency to provide the energy to sustain your vital functions such as the liver, heart, kidneys, brain, skeletal and muscle, and maintain regulatory balance at rest. This can be referred to as your Resting Metabolic Rate; it is an ideal base to construct any kind of weight management plan, which may include calorie restriction, physical activity, or ideally both.

There are several factors, which can affect your Resting Metabolic Rate, including:

- muscle mass;   having more muscle will increase it
- climate;   cold conditions will increase it
- eating;   regular and less quantity meals will increase it
- supplements;   some supplements can raise it (not advised)
- pregnancy;   will increase it
- extreme dieting;   will decrease it
- aging;   getting older (from 20 onwards) will decrease it

What is your Resting Metabolic Rate?
The Resting Metabolic Rate formula will give you the answer and it is the same formula for both men and women, firstly:

1. Using your body fat percentage (which you need to have measured) and total body weight (kg), workout the weight of your fat in kilograms

2. Subtract the kilograms of body fat from your total body weight; the resulting figure is your fat-free body mass

3. Multiply your fat-free body mass (kg) by the number **30** in the Resting Metabolic Rate formula

For example,

Step 1	Total body weight			70kg x (multiply)
	Your body fat %			20%
			=	14kg body fat
Step 2	70kg	-	14kg =	__56kg__ fat-free body mass
Step3	56kg	x	30 =	__1,680 kcal__ Resting Metabolic Rate

Tony, from the example above, is an average person of 70kg with a fat percentage of 20%; and he will need approximately 1,680 calories to fulfil his Resting Metabolic Rate just to sustain life. Angela, a 60kg woman with a medium / high fat percentage (30%) will require 1,260 calories: 60kg – 18kg (60kg x 30%) = 42kg; 42kg x 30 = 1,260 kcal per day. While Sanjay, on the other hand, is overweight, weighing 80kg of which is 30% body fat: 80kg – 24kg (80kg x 30%) = 56kg; 56kg x 30 = 1,680 kcal per day.

Look at the Resting Metabolic Rates of Tony and Sanjay. They are both the same; Sanjay has the Resting Metabolic Rate of 1,680 as does Tony; this is because the Resting Metabolic Rate, which sustains the vital functions at rest, only takes into account the fat-free mass of a person.

Your Resting Metabolic Rate is:

Step 1	Total body weight			____kg x (multiply)
	Your body fat %			____%
			=	____kg body fat
Step 2	______kg	-	______kg =	______kg fat-free body mass
Step3	______kg	x	30 =	______kcal Resting Metabolic Rate

What is your Total Energy Expenditure?
The next stage is to work out your daily Total Energy Expenditure

1. Take your Resting Metabolic Rate and multiply it by the figure, which best describes your activity level taken from the table below:

Activity level guideline for general populations

	Men	Women
Sedentary (inactive)	1.1	1.1
Lightly Active (e.g. office workers)	1.2	1.15
Moderately active (e.g. light industrial)	1.3	1.25
Very active (e.g. builders)	1.4	1.35
Exceptionally active*	*should seek the advice of a Nutritionalist	

E.g.,   Tony is an office worker and his activity level is **1.2**.

1,680kcal	x	1.2	= 2,016 kcal per day
Resting Metabolic Rate		activity level	

Your Total Energy Expenditure is:

______ kcal	x	____	= ______ kcal per day
Resting Metabolic Rate		activity level	

Now that you have worked out your Resting Metabolic Rate and Total Energy Expenditure, you can unlock the secrets to perfect bodyweight management. Raising your Resting Metabolic Rate by increasing your muscle mass (see Chapter 17 – Activity for life) and by eating smaller and regular meals (see Chapter 10 – Food for thought) you can also fight the effects of aging, and be empowered to better health and longevity.

Remember that when you are:

- in excess of your Total Energy Rate; you will increase in bodyweight, as the unutilised calories are converted to fat or be wasted
- below your Total Energy Expenditure **but** above your Resting Metabolic Rate you will lose weight gradually and safely
- below your Total Energy Expenditure **and** below your Resting Metabolic Rate, you will:
  - lose weight initially
  - start hinder your body functions
  - decrease your Resting Metabolic Rate (to match your calorie intake)
  - stop losing weight

Crash dieters beware!
If you were to go on a diet of 1,000 calories (and your Resting Metabolic Rate is 1,500 calories), you will initially lose weight; then reach a plateau

and stop losing it. Furthermore, when you eventually resume eating as normal (not a choice, but a question of survival) you will put the lost weight back on, and on most occasions, rise past your original body weight.

To reduce your intake to 1,000 calories per day (while your Resting Metabolic Rate is a higher figure) will put your body in to a 'starvation stress' situation. It will respond by reducing the efficiency of your internal organs and muscles, and in doing so reduce the energy you require to function. You will lose weight until your body adjusts to the stress the diet is causing it and until it matches the 1,000 calories, you are supplying it to survive. It is here you will reach a plateau. If you notice that you have stopped losing weight and try to reduce the calories further, your body will keep reducing your vital body functions to match the calories you are supplying it. As you continue to reduce the calorie intake, so the body continues to reduce the body functions, and you will experience dizzy spells, lethargy, fainting, and such like. This is a vicious circle taking you down a path of danger and life threatening consequences. You will have to restore your food intake to above your Resting Metabolic Rate; otherwise, your body will shut you down!

Food choices
The food choices you make will directly affect and determine your quality of life. The immediate impact of foods you eat can range from pleasurable sensations to lethargy, from hyperactivity to mental alertness and mood enhancing. How many people have had the misfortune to experience the feeling of lethargy and sleepiness after having eaten and drunk a little too much at one sitting. Is in not the case that following this kind of overindulgence your energy levels are drained so much that you feel unable to move and eventually succumb to an unplanned snooze or nap. On the other hand, how about the buzz or heady sensation you feel after having enjoyed your favourite food. For most people, their favourite foods revolve around sugary (and fat) related items. After all, your instincts have been programmed this way to ensure human survival for the previous thousands of years.

The mid-term effects of your nutrition will increase or decrease your quality of health. You can be empowered by increased energy levels, uplifted moods, super efficient body functions, strengthened immune system, and increased mental capacity. Alternatively, be plagued by fatigue, irritability, cravings, mood swings, lapses in memory or concentration, headaches, difficulties in sleeping lacking motivation, and suffer issues such as food allergies, sensitivities, skin ailments, bad breath, faulty digestion, water retention, appetite disruptions, and dental problems.

The longer term effects of poor nutrition can lead you from illness to disease; there are many leading scientists working in this field and have produced numerous studies to support the fact that a ill conceived diet can lead to diseases such as obesity, diabetes type-2, some cancers, osteoporosis, high blood pressure, coronary artery disease, and stroke. It causes millions of premature deaths, uncountable days of pain and suffering, and costs billions in health care. This has led to all sorts of professionals, officials, groups, industries, organisations, and governments to seek solutions to these problems, and try their best to control the risk factors with their own (mostly biased) nutritional advice.

Nuts and bolts
To summarize, the human body needs energy in order to sustain life and the food you eat is the source of this energy. It is the base from which, your biological and chemical reactions are initiated; also, the repairing and renewing functions of the body use this food energy to do their work. The food you eat is broken down to its smallest elements and this chemical reaction releases the energy which sustains body functions, such as respiration, brain signals, circulation, thermoregulation, as well as during rest and when physically active. Food consists of various nutrients and these can initially be divided into macronutrients and micronutrients. The macronutrients are the carbohydrates, fats, proteins, and fibre (fibre is normally grouped in with the carbohydrates but is significant enough to warrant separate detailing).

Macronutrients	**Micro**nutrients
Carbohydrates	Vitamins
Fibre	Minerals
Protein	
Fats	

Carbohydrates and fats (and in rare situations proteins) provide you with energy; protein and minerals form the building blocks for repair; and vitamins, minerals, and fats facilitate chemical reactions to move muscle and your metabolism. Some foods are bursting with nutrients providing enormous value to the body, while others can supply energy, and carry no nutritional value at all. Filling your body with too much or too little nutrients will lead to a body malfunction and ultimately illness or disease; your body needs to have the optimum balance of nutrients to maintain perfect health. As you can see it is vital to understand how the food you eat and the nutrients they provide help you achieve the perfect balance.

The Macronutrients
Carbohydrates - Not all carbohydrates are equal
Carbohydrates protect and help preserve protein tissue, facilitate the body's breakdown of fat, and supply the brain and red blood cells with energy. Carbohydrates can be separated into two broad sections: Simple carbohydrates (sugars) which come in two forms, monosaccharide, & disaccharide such as glucose, sucrose, fructose, maltose, and lactose, and complex carbohydrates, which are polysaccharides and can be separated into starch, a digestible complex carbohydrate, and fibre, an indigestible one such as seeds, corn, grains, cereal, pasta, peas, potatoes, and root vegetables.

The average person will consume between 45 to 55% of total calories from carbohydrates. In recent times, that figure remains the same, despite high protein diets and such like. The change has been seen in what carbohydrates people choose to eat. People are more likely to get their carbohydrates from simple sugars now as oppose to the complex ones they used to eat. Twenty years ago, a person's yearly intake of sugar was 57g, today it is over 71g, a rise of over 25%. Foods and drinks, which have been processed with added sugar, have benefited the most, as they are consumed by the million; fizzy drinks with twelve teaspoons of sugar in a can; or fruit flavoured yoghurts with seven teaspoons. Unlike the sugars associated with fruit, added sugars only provide energy (calories) and no added nutrients; these types of added sugar are referred to as 'empty' calories.

> To find these 'empty' calories in food; look out for ingredients such as sugar, brown sugar, raw sugar, corn syrup, corn-syrup solids, high-fructose corn syrup, malt, syrup, maple syrup, pancake syrup, fructose sweetener, liquid fructose, honey, molasses, anhydrous dextrose, and crystal dextrose.
>
> *Health-Warrior*

It is easy to classify the carbohydrates into simple and complex, however, the effects on the body are a little more difficult to group. All the carbohydrates (excluding fibre), simple or complex will, after consumption, be broken down into glucose and raise your blood glucose (also known as blood sugar) and insulin levels. The extent of how much your blood glucose level rises after eating a specific carbohydrate, is measured by the Glycemic Index. There have been many diet books and countless articles based solely on the Glycemic Index number of foods. They correctly identified that low Glycemic Index foods produce only relatively smaller fluctuations in your blood glucose and insulin levels. However, this is a very basic approach to a more complex situation. The

Glycemic Load concept was developed by scientists to describe the quality (Glycemic Index) and quantity of carbohydrate in a meal or diet.

The rise and the fall

Your body will always look to remain in a balanced state; and the balancing of your blood glucose and insulin levels is no different. Ideally, you should have small rises in blood glucose and insulin levels after food intake, and fall slightly below normal a few hours later to initiate the hunger trigger. Foods that have a high Glycemic Load will produce a rapid rise in the space of a few minutes in your blood glucose level; to counteract this rapid rise, insulin is released into your blood stream. This rapid rise sparks a rapid fall in the body blood glucose level. The rapid fall leads to feelings of lethargy, cravings, headaches, and irritability. To make matters worse, as your body is trying to regain balance in glucose levels, you may react by consuming a sugar snack, fizzy drink, chocolate bar, tea, or coffee. You may feel better for a brief period, but this rapid rise will again be quickly followed by another fall. This fall is caused by your body releasing the hormone insulin into your blood stream, to get the excess glucose out and into the body cells for use as energy, or if not used, to be stored as fat.

This is a vicious circle and the short-term symptoms are:

- fatigue
- irritability
- extra snacking in between meals
- cravings for sweet foods / drinks
- lack of motivation, concentration, memory
- excess sweating
- sleep and relaxation problems
- headaches
- constant craving for coffee / tea / cigarette

The physical response of your body to high glucose levels and excessive insulin are:

- impaired glucose tolerance
- insulin resistance
- increased serum triglyceride concentrations
- decreased high density lipoproteins or HDL cholesterol
  - HDL cholesterol is considered good cholesterol, because higher blood levels of HDL cholesterol are associated with lower risk of heart disease.

The health illnesses and diseases, which have been associated with these kinds of body adaptations, are:

> **Diabetes** - High blood glucose levels and excessive insulin secretion contribute to the loss of the insulin-secreting function of your body and leads to irreversible diabetes. The foods that were most consistently associated with increased risk of type 2 diabetes were potatoes, white rice, white bread, and carbonated beverages. Low Glycemic Load food plans improved short-term and long-term control of blood glucose levels in people with type 1 and 2 diabetes.

> **Obesity** - Is a major risk factor for developing type 2 diabetes, in fact, 97% of all cases of type 2 diabetes are cause by excess weight. According to the Centres for Disease Control and Prevention in the United States, type 2 diabetes has tripled in the last 30 years, largely due to the global epidemic of obesity. Studies have shown that a low Glycemic Load food plan will reduce weight in obese people. In a review of published studies David Ludwig of Harvard Medical School, found that fifteen out of sixteen studies concluded that low Glycemic Load foods delayed the hunger sensation, decreased subsequent intake, and increased 'the full' feeling, when compared with high Glycemic Load foods.

> **Cardiovascular disease** - High blood glucose levels and excessive insulin secretion leads to irreversible diabetes. Furthermore, people who suffer type 2 diabetes also increase the risk of cardiovascular disease and are 2 to 4 times at greater risk than people without diabetes, to suffer a heart disease or stroke.

> **Cancer** - In separate studies, conducted in Canada and the United States, it was found that high Glycemic index foods increased the risk of colon and breast cancer (especially those who reported no physical activity).

The Glycemic Load: a closer look; the GL Factor
The Glycemic Load is the way to assess the impact of carbohydrate consumption, which takes account of the Glycemic Index and empowers you to make better choices than just looking at the Glycemic Index number alone. The Glycemic Index number of a food lets you know how rapidly it will be turned into sugar. The Glycemic Load value tells you how much carbohydrate is available in that food and calculates more accurately how quickly the food will increase your blood sugar levels. In

essence, each unit of the Glycemic Load represents the equivalent blood sugar-raising effect of 1 gram of pure glucose.

Glycemic Load 20 or more	High
11 to 19	Medium
10 or less	Low

Most of the time, foods which have a low Glycemic Load value have a low Glycemic Index one, where as foods with medium or high Glycemic Loads range in value from very low to very high Glycemic index values. This is where knowledge and use of the Glycemic Load values will help you reduce the risk of heart disease, diabetes, and obesity. Daily dietary Glycemic Index has been found to be positively associated to your body weight fat percentage and follows the proven theory that increased Glycemic Index foods result in more insulin being produced and more fat being stored. Researchers have also found that lowering and adjusting the type of carbohydrate, and lowering the Glycemic Load has resulted in the weight loss of research participants. For example, instant white rice on the Glycemic Index is listed as having a value of 46 and is recognised as at the low end of the scale, and implies that the effect on your blood sugar levels will be relatively moderate. However, instant rice has a large carbohydrate content, and on the Glycemic Load scale, it tips into the high category, indicating a bigger impact on your blood sugar level. Instant white rice may have a medium Glycemic Index rating but because it has more carbohydrate in it, it has a higher impact on your blood sugar level.

On the other hand, the carbohydrate in watermelon, for instance, has a high Glycemic Index (72). However, there is not a lot of carbohydrate in it, as it is mostly water, so watermelon's Glycemic Load is relatively low. According to the calculations by the people at the University of Sydney's Human Nutrition Unit, in a serving of 120 grams it has six grams of available carbohydrate per serving, so its Glycemic Load is low, at about four. Below there are examples of the action and effects of when you eat foods with different Glycemic Load values.

The **action** is followed by the **effect** on your blood sugar levels:

Action : Eat foods higher than Glycemic Load 20
Effect   : Rapid rise in minutes - followed by rapid fall

Action : Drink sugary drinks / concentrated fruit juice
Effect   : Rapid rise in minutes - followed by rapid fall

Action : Drink caffeine / alcohol
Effect   : Rapid rise in minutes - followed by rapid fall

Action : Missing meals (or gaps of longer than 5 hours)
Effect   : Glucose level falls - glucose is taken out of blood circulation -
initiating intense cravings for sugar such as sweet foods / drinks

Now you understand the negative effects of continually eating high Glycemic Load foods to your health, you can make a better-informed and healthier choice: The '**informed action**' is followed by the **effect** on your blood sugar levels:

Informed action: Foods eaten with Glycemic Load rating of less than 20
Effect   : Rise gradually over a few hours and adopt a measured return to normal

Informed action: Meals eaten regularly
Effect   : Rise and falls gradually over a few hours

Informed action: Gaps between meals and / or snacks no longer then four hours
Effect   : This will reduce wild swings in your blood sugar levels.

Informed action: Portions sizes kept to small and medium
Effect   : Blood sugar levels will rise and fall gradually over a few hours

Food combinations

> The larger the carbohydrate contents of the meal, the greater the Glycemic Load, and therefore the bigger influences on your blood sugar levels and insulin.
>
> *Health-Warrior*

The effect of combining foods on your blood sugar levels is a straightforward matter. In the most recent of studies conducted at the Institute of Nutrition and Food Technology (INTA), it concluded that the carbohydrate content of food accounts for 90% of the blood sugar and insulin responses of the body. It showed that protein and fat portions of the meals made little contributions to the blood sugar and insulin responses. You would be wasting your time, and could be adversely affecting your health if you thought that mixing your meals, by adding protein or fat, would somehow reduce the effect on your blood sugar or insulin levels. This is a key finding affecting your future health, and below are some examples of Glycemic Load food values. Look up the resources section in the back of this book your will find the websites with Glycemic Index and Load values for most foods.

Food	Glycemic Load per serving	Glycemic Index	Serving size
Pears, raw	4	38	1 medium
Lentils, dried; boiled	5	29	1 cup
Rye, pumpernickel bread	5	41	1 large slice
Oranges, raw	5	42	1 medium
Apples, raw	6	38	1 medium
Kidney beans, dried; boiled	7	28	1 cup
Table sugar	7	68	2 tsp
White bread	10	73	1 large slice
Barley; boiled	11	25	1 cup
Spaghetti, whole wheat; boiled	14	37	1 cup
Doughnut	17	76	1 medium
Puffed rice cakes	17	78	3 cakes
Brown rice (boiled)	18	55	1 cup
Cornflakes	21	81	1 cup
White rice (boiled)	23	64	1 cup
Baked potato	23	76	1 medium
Pancake	39	67	6" diameter
Dates, dried	42	103	60g

The Glycemic Load is for carbohydrates

Do not be lured into the trap into thinking ALL foods with low Glycemic Loads are 'good' foods. The benefits of the Glycemic Load can only be used to any effect on foods, which have a majority of carbohydrate content. When it comes to foods with high protein or fat content you have to look at them as separate from the Glycemic Index and Glycemic Load scales.

For example, all the following foods have super Glycemic Load readings of less than one: strawberry shortcake, sausages, and vanilla ice cream (their Glycemic Index values are 42, 28, and 32 respectively). The majority of calories from these foods, come from the mixture of fat, protein, and sugar, and only when you look at the fat, protein, sugar, and salt components can you really determine the quality of the food and its positive or negative health impacts. A working knowledge of the general foods you eat and the effect they have on your blood glucose levels, will give you greater control over your good health.

Use this knowledge and you can look forward to:

- control over your weight, losing it where necessary
- reduced hunger attacks and keeping you satisfied for longer
- positive sensitivity to insulin and greater diabetes control
- reduce the risk of heart disease and lower blood cholesterol levels
- more energy over longer periods of time

Here are 3 golden rules to follow and reap the benefits immediately:

1. Try to eat foods that have Glycemic Load ratings of less than 15 (ideally aiming for less than 10)

2. Increasing the consumption of whole grains, nuts, legumes, fruits and non-starchy vegetables

3. Do not miss meals and keep portion sizes small to medium

In addition, try to reduce the burdens to your body blood glucose balance by avoiding:

- coffee and tea
- alcohol and cigarettes
- extreme high sugar foods (such as honey, jams, and syrup)
- refined processed foods (such as white bread, rice, cookies, cakes, candy and soft-drinks)
- fruit juice / dried fruit on their own (eat the fruit instead it's so much better for you)

Fabulous fibre – A complex carbohydrate
It has a complex structure, it is a non-starch, found exclusively in plant cells and walls, and is indigestible. It includes cellulose, which is the most plentiful organic molecule in the world. Fibre is further split into two groups:

Water-soluble fibre:
One of its major roles is to lower blood cholesterol levels. Good sources of soluble fibre include fruits, vegetables, oat bran, barley, seed husks, flaxseed, beans, lentils, peas, soymilk and soy products.

Insoluble fibre:
A major role of insoluble fibre is to add bulk to faeces and to prevent constipation and associated problems such as haemorrhoids. Good sources include wheat bran, corn bran, rice bran, the skins of fruits and vegetables, nuts, seeds, dried beans, and wholegrain foods.

These structures belong to the complex carbohydrates and will resist breakdown and pass through the body without producing any energy at all. Both types of fibre are beneficial to the body and most plant foods contain a mixture of both types. There are many positive health impacts of a high fibre intake, and have been linked to lower cases of obesity, diabetes, digestive disorders, some cancers, and heart disease. Fibre will reduce the insulin secreted by the body by slowing down the nutrient absorption after a meal. Fibre content also decreases the total number of calories consumed in subsequent meals. In a study published in the American Journal of Clinical Nutrition, it was found that a high fibre cereal breakfast reduced the buffet style meal eaten at lunch when compared to participants who had eaten a low fibre breakfast. The medical centre in Minneapolis, United States, also reported that participants did not feel less hungry, even though they consumed fewer calories.

Just by increasing your fibre intake into your daily food plan, you can start to lose significant amounts of excess body fat. High fibre foods are more filling and are mostly lower fat lower calorie, you will also need to chew a little longer and this contributes to a greater feeling of 'food satisfaction'. The slowing of the digestive system allows you to feel 'full' for longer and prevents any rapid rises in blood sugar levels.

Fibre and its effects on certain illness and diseases:

Dampening diabetes - The high fibre in complex carbohydrates reduces the rapid rises in blood sugar and insulin levels; this slowing of the glucose absorption into the blood stream allows people with a risk of diabetes to prevent or control the onset of the disease.

Efficient digestion - A high fibre food plan keeps your digestive system in perfect working order. Keeping your body hydrated by drinking adequate amounts of water will be required to 'lubricate' the fibre on its journey. As you age, the slower your digestive system operates and this makes fibre and water even more important to your good health.

Reduce your cholesterol - A food plan, which includes oat bran, beans, and soybeans, have been proven to reduce cholesterol levels. This is turn will help reduce the risks of coronary heart disease by decreasing the fatty and plaque deposits on your artery walls and prevent blood flow through your artery passages from being impeded.

Can it help fight cancer?
Fibre in food items such as fruits, vegetables, and cereals has been shown to reduce the risks of some cancers (such as mouth, throat, and stomach). Fibre holds considerable amounts of water and it has been suggested that their scraping action along the gut wall and the absorption and hindrance of harmful chemicals on route, help to reduce the body's exposure to cancer causing carcinogens.

How to increase your fibre intake

Fibre is mostly lost when food is processed and cooked.
Health-Warrior

- Eat a high fibre breakfast cereals that contain barley, wheat or oats
- Eat wholemeal, multigrain breads and brown rice
- Read the labels! Do not rely on package advertising to make your choice
    - High fibre 5 g or more per serving;
    - Good fibre 2.5 g to 4.9 g per serving;
    - Average fibre 1.5g to 2.5 g per serving
- Eat your fruit and vegetables raw
- Snack on fruit, vegetables, and nuts

Here is a list of fibre content in common foods:

Serving size	Fibre	Grams
Breads, cereals, grains		
Whole grain bread	1 slice	1.7
Oatmeal, cooked	1 cup	4.0
Rice, brown, cooked	1 cup	3.5
Fruit		
Apple, with skin	1 large	3.3
Blackberries	1 cup	7.6
Orange	1 small	3.1
Pear	1 med	5.1
Strawberries	1 cup	3.3

Vegetables

Kidney beans	1 cup	9.0
Beans, green, cooked	1 cup	4.0
Broccoli, raw	1 cup	2.3
Cabbage, raw	1 cup	1.6
Carrots, raw	1 cup	3.1
Lentils, cooked	1/2 cup	8.3
Peas, boiled	1 cup	4.5
Tomato, red, ripe	1 tomato	1.5

Nuts

| Almonds | 12 nuts | 1.7 |

Protein

The word 'protein' comes from the Greek word 'protas' meaning 'of primary importance'. It is a complex organic compound and is involved in practically every function performed by a cell in the human body. It is essential to the structure of red blood cells, for the proper functioning of antibodies resisting infection, for the regulation of enzymes and hormones, for growth, and for the repair of body tissue. Basically, the collection of muscles, bones, skin, blood, tissue, cells, genes, and such like is made-up from the building blocks of protein; where your body composition minus the without the water content is 75% protein. Protein is made from the elements carbon, hydrogen, oxygen, and importantly, nitrogen, which is used to determine the protein content of a food.

There is a 'new' you everyday

There are thousands of different protein structure combinations and they are constantly being renewed; out with the old structures and in with the new ones. Your body structures are being replaced everyday and during the course of a year, almost all of your body has been renewed!

> When it comes to slowing down the ageing process and enhancing overall health, no food is more important than protein.
>
> *Lesley Kenton*
> *Age Power*

Meet the Amino Acids

When protein is eaten, it is first broken down into peptides (linked amino acids), and further broken down in to amino acids. There are, at last count, 22 amino acids, which are the basic building blocks of protein, 9 are essential, and the other 13 non-essential. The nine essential amino acids are histidine, isoleucine, leucine, lysine, methionine, phenylalanine, threonine, tryptophan, and valine. They are deemed essential because they cannot be synthesized by the body in the amounts needed, and are therefore essential to healthy nutrition. For those who do not eat meat, fish, eggs, or dairy products, it is important to eat a variety of plant origin sources of protein, in order to get the full compliment of these essential amino acids. Though plant foods contain the same nine essential amino acids as animal food sources do, they do not, (with the exception of some soy products), contain all nine in the one food or in the quantities, the animal sources do.

However, this should not be regarded as a negative situation, because in fact, it forces you to consume a variety of different foods in order to fulfil your essential amino acids quota.

> Look in the appendix section at the back of this book to discover the 'Plant origin sources of the 9 Essential Amino Acids'.
>
> *Health-Warrior*

Furthermore, new research has shown that it is no longer a requirement, as previously believed, to eat the complete range of essential amino acids at the same meal. For example, previous advice on vegetarian websites would talk of 'protein combining' in the same meal in order to ensure all essential amino acids were consumed; meal combinations such as, beans on multigrain toast, a peanut butter sandwich, muesli with soy milk, and brown rice with peas or beans are good examples of such. The benefits of consuming a plant source for your protein oppose to an animal based one are reduced risks of diseases such as obesity, coronary artery disease, hypertension, diabetes, and some types of cancer. Moreover, you can look forward to a boosted immune system, and lower saturated fat and cholesterol intake. The majority of the world's protein consumption is derived from plant foods, of which cereals are by far the most important. There are noteworthy geographical differences.

Throughout the developed world, animal sources provide the majority of protein intake, whereas in developing countries cereals are the number one source. The factors affecting these global differences can be attributed to the cost of protein, household income (the higher the income the more likely to consume animal protein), environment, and religion.

> Although human beings eat meat, we are not natural carnivores. No matter how much fat carnivores [in the animal world] eat, they do not develop atherosclerosis [clogged up arteries].
>
> *Dr WC Roberts*
> *Editor-In-Chief, American Journal of Cardiology*

Meat is undoubtedly a rich source of protein and has all the necessary essential amino acids in one portion, but in excess quantities has a negative impact on your health. The issue is that the protein source (including dairy products) comes mixed with saturated fat and cholesterol. Increased intake of saturated fat and cholesterol will elevate your risk of suffering from obesity, heart disease, hypertension, diabetes, some types of cancer, and a weakened immune system.

Protein sources

Animal origin sources - Complete proteins (those that contain **all** the essential amino acids): Meat, milk, cheese, and egg

Plant origin sources -   Incomplete proteins (contain some of the essential amino acids) such as whole grains, bread, rice, corn, beans, legumes, oatmeal, peas, and nuts, and soya products

> The quality of protein is compromised when it is cooked; foods like meat, fish, poultry, eggs, and milk lose some of the essential amino acids in the process, rendering them incomplete.
>
> *Health-Warrior*

What should my protein intake be?

The scientists are still not certain as to the optimum daily intake of protein. The World Health Organisation claims it should be 10 to 15% of your total daily calories. Nutrition experts claim 10 to 12%, while the United Kingdom Department of health and the United States Food and Nutrition Board both recommend for both men and women is 0.80 g of good quality protein per kilogram of body weight per day (which also works out to between 10 to 12% for most people). The best way to calculate your daily protein needs are using the daily protein calculator below (noting that you will need to use 12% for your protein quota if you are vegan or vegetarian). To compete the protein calculator, you need to work out your Total Energy Expenditure (refer back to p.63).

Your daily protein requirement calculator

Step 1   Total Energy Expenditure _________________x (*multiply by*)

Your protein quota _______________%

= ______________kcal

Step 2   (*divide by*) /   __4___

=   _______grams (daily protein requirement)

For example,

Step 1   Total Energy Expenditure   __2,016 kcal__ x (*multiply by*)

Your protein quota ________10________%

= ________201________kcal

Step 2   (*divide by*) / ____4____

=   ____50____ grams (daily protein requirement)

Most people are looking at a daily protein intake of between 45g and 65g depending on age, weight, state of health, and other factors. A lack of protein can make you tired and lethargic; you will tend to feel colder than others and have trouble concentrating. You could be susceptible to increased blood glucose with its negative health impacts. In addition, aesthetically you could be looking in the mirror at increasing amounts of greying hair, losing tone in your muscles, and a few more wrinkles than for your age. Your attitude might not be much better as you may suffer mood swings, loss of muscle mass, low body temperature, hormonal irregularities, as well as loss of skin elasticity.

An average person would not have too much trouble achieving the recommended daily allowance. For example, below highlights the protein elements of a diet with average portion sizes, and this achieves the recommended daily allowance:

Breakfast

A nut and seed rich muesli, milk, and two slices of whole grain toast.

Lunch

Sausage or tofu sandwich

Dinner

Brown rice, peas, chicken

Protein deficiency does not seem to be a problem for developing countries, for example, the United Kingdom, where population surveys of British adults showed that the average daily protein intake for men was 84g and for women it was 64g. That is far over the recommended daily allowances.

Is too much protein a health hazard?

Most diets provide more protein than the body needs, with the excess coming from animal sources, causing excess nitrogen to be excreted in urine. The excess nitrogen has been linked in some studies with reduced kidney function in old age. Too much protein intake can cause damage to your bone density; caused by the increase in calcium removed from your body; linking high-protein (particularly animal protein) diets with osteoporosis.

Allergies and protein

The structure of each protein compound is slightly different, and this difference can cause the immune system to dysfunction, while others pass by perfectly safely. This immune system dysfunction can trigger allergic reactions in some people. Can you think of someone you know who has a food allergy? Most people can. In most cases, people are allergic to everyday foods such as milk protein (casein), wheat and other grain proteins (gluten), peanuts, or seafood. Do you know of anyone who as adverse allergic reactions to **more than** one of these foods? This is very rare indeed.

The powder proteins

There is a whole new industry been created by first the athletes and body builders, but now being used by the public to supply their protein needs. It is the protein-powder supplement industry and its commercially manufactured proteins. The main types of protein powder are:

- whey protein isolate and whey protein concentrate are both produced from whey (a by-product of cheese making)
- soy protein isolate

These versions of the protein powder are a little older and less used:

- milk protein is made up of about 80% casein and 20% whey protein
- egg white protein - spray dried egg whites are used in some 'egg and milk' protein powder mixes

Whey proteins and soy proteins have been trumpeted as the 'perfect' proteins, the 21st century way to absorb them into your body. The measure of protein quality is its Biological Value, and it is based on a scale, which relates to the retention and absorption into the body. On the scale the higher the number is the better the retention and absorption; for example, rice has the value of 59, an egg 100, and whey protein isolates up to 159. It is facts like these that have helped create the millions of sales worldwide. They recommend its daily use, as a snack, liquid meals, or as an added ingredient to a normal meal; using the argument that a higher quality protein will allow your body to make better use of it than if it were consumed as a meat, fish or plant source.

The protein powders are artificially engineered foods and they can be made fat free and boosted by added vitamins and minerals. However, these multi-coloured powders are no match for the taste, variety, or the derived pleasures of real food.

In a study in Holland, human growth was measured over a 3-year period using natural proteins and substitute ones. The natural protein was shown to improve the growth in the subjects over the 3-year period, whereas the substitute did not.

Leave the powder to the scientists!

How to maximise your protein intake and usage:

- Eat a protein source at every meal
- Eat mostly plant proteins - avoiding excess saturated fat and cholesterol in animal sources; (Otherwise, highest quality fish, chicken, and low fat dairy products are good choices from the animal sources).
- Increase the variety of you protein sources (and get all the essential amino acids)
- Minimise cooking times (e.g. steam or soak beans and legumes for 24 hrs; in fresh in season vegetables such as broad beans or green peas can be used without cooking, for example, in salads)
- Avoid pre-packaged, processed, and 'added to' food items – there are big reductions in ALL nutrients in these foods and will most probably contain high trans fats, salt, and sugar
- Avoid manufactured proteins, such as powders, bars, and meal replacements

Fats & Oils

Fats are made up of the elements carbon, hydrogen, and (small amounts of oxygen). The basic unit of fat is a triglyceride with fatty acids and glycerol its building blocks. Fats are usually divided into two groups: saturated and unsaturated (monounsaturated and polyunsaturated).

Relatively, new additional groups can also be added to the two above: the new hybrid of fats, the manufactured trans-fatty acids, and the much talked about derived fats, cholesterol. As the following pages will reveal, there are clear distinctions between all the groupings, and each elicits different influences on your good health and optimum body functioning.

Fat, the fall guy

Whether you like it or not, you need fat, and it is essential to overall good health and to vital body functions. Fats in general have been focused on extensively by governments, organisations, associations, food industry, media, and the health industry in general, and you are constantly being advised to reduce your fat intake. This very general 'one-size-fits-all' advice is inaccurate and can cause serious problems in the body, where fat is severely restricted from the diet. Fats are the most concentrated source of energy at nine calories per gram of fat, available to you. Studies prove that excess fat consumption is a major cause of obesity and is a major risk factor in diseases such as, high blood pressure, coronary heart disease, and colon cancer. Are there fats, which can help you avoid illness and disease?

Fat has little impact on your blood glucose and insulin levels, and it has been proven to decrease your appetite; its important body functions include:

- energy storage and supply
- protection of vital organs
- thermal insulation
- transporters of vitamins
- facilitates communication to brain (e.g. hunger suppressant)

A fat-free diet is an unhealthy one; choose your fats wisely and you will reap the rewards of increased good health. In a study published in the New England Journal of Medicine, assessing the risk of coronary heart disease and fat intake, reported that a reduction of 5% saturated fatty acids, which was replaced by mono- or poly- unsaturated fatty acids reduced the coronary heart disease risk by 42%. To fully appreciate how fat is vital to well-being and how these health problems relate to fat and its consumption, it is important to understand the different types of fat you consume and the ways they affect you.

> Remember all fats in food contain a mixture of fatty acids, but one type tends to dominate in that food; such as, beef will be predominantly saturated or corn oil will predominantly be polyunsaturated.
>
> *Health-Warrior*

Saturated fats or fatty acids

A saturated fatty acid is jammed full of hydrogen and carbon atoms with no empty places for this compound to join with other substances. They can be found in animal products (such as beef, veal, lamb, pork, and ham), dairy produce (such as whole milk, cream, cheese, and egg yolk), vegetable by-products (such as coconut oil, palm oil, and shortening), and prepared foods (such as cakes, pies, cookies, snacks, and fast foods). For an average person with a food intake of 2,000 kcal, it is recommended not to consume more than 5% or 11 grams of saturated fats. Bearing in mind a doughnut (saturated fat 3.2g), medium sized portion of French fries (saturated fat 6.8g), and a glass of whole milk (saturated fat 1g) fulfils the recommended level in just one meal!

> Even pet food is healthier for you than fast foods such as
> KFC chicken pieces, McDonalds Big Mac, or a Pizza
> Hut pizza, as it contains less fat, salt, and sugar!
>
> *Source: The Sunday Times*

In the days of 'feast or famine', saturated fatty acids may have provided a high-energy source, which was stored in the feast phase with the purpose of being used in the famine phase. In modern times, there are no good reasons for consumption of saturated fatty acids, as they offer no benefits to health and are not necessary to the human body (unlike their counterparts the unsaturated fatty acids which can fulfil all the requirements of the human body and more). In fact, consumption of saturated fatty acids have been shown to cause significant increases in 'bad' cholesterol, which can lead to diseases such as heart disease.

> Always read the food labels – a quick 10-second scan of
> the food is all it takes – your health, wellness, and
> longevity are at stake.
>
> *Health-Warrior*

Polyunsaturated fatty acids (Essential fatty acids)
Polyunsaturated fatty acids are also known as essential fatty acids because they are needed for your body to function. They can be further separated into omega-3 and omega-6 fatty acids, and without them, you would not be able to operate efficiently, as they support the structure and offer protection of the brain, eyes, ears, reproductive organs, skin and much more. They are also used in hormone-like production, essential for cellular functions, immune system, reproductive functions, central nervous system, and of course, the heart and brain.

In a recent study, a component of omega-3 has been identified to provide anti-inflammatory effects on a person's joints and to improve blood circulation and flow. It was shown to work by inhibiting the production and regulating the migration of inflammatory cells and chemicals to sites of inflammation; a natural cure for a common ailment. Unlike the unnatural use of anti-inflammatory drugs, such as aspirin and ibuprofen, omega-3 inhibitors do not have negative side effects on the gastrointestinal or cardiovascular systems.

Omega-3: A wonder nutrient, what it can do for you
Sources: Flaxseed (linseed), pumpkin seeds, walnuts, hemp seeds, soybeans and some dark green leafy vegetables, corn oil, safflower oil, sunflower oil, and canola oil. Cold-water fish including salmon, tuna, halibut, and herring

Essential omega-3 can
- reduce inflammation throughout your body
- lessen and inhibit any excessive blood clotting
- promote excellent blood flow throughout your body
- ensure you body cells operate efficiently and despatch waste from your body
- lower your cholesterol levels
- improve the body's ability to respond to insulin helps regulate food intake, body weight and metabolism
- reduce the risk of becoming obese

Essential omega-3 can also help in the fight against conditions and symptoms such as:
- depression
- cardiovascular disease
- type 2 diabetes
- fatigue
- dry, itchy skin
- brittle hair and nails
- ability to concentrate and focus
- joint pain

Omega-6: Making you look younger and stay healthier
Sources: Vegetable oils: rapeseed, sunflower, etc and Evening primrose and starflower oil

Look younger, with glowing skin, fewer wrinkles, vibrant hair, and nails; these are what omega-6 can offer you. It uses its anti-inflammatory and rejuvenating talents, to empower your body cells and skin layers to resist the effects of aging and the general wear and tear of modern life. Forget all those creams and chemicals, omega-6 your 'beauty' nutrient will help you fight the symptoms such as
- pale and inelastic skin
- dry skin and scalp
- limp and lifeless hair
- brittle nails

In addition, to helping you stay younger, in keeps you healthier for longer and will:

- master the hormone balance; and relieves symptoms such as premenstrual tension (PMT) in women
- boost your immune system
- put fluidity back into joints

Omega-6 attacks arthritis

Studies show that omega-6 used long-term will achieve the maximum benefits, for instance many arthritis patients reported that their joints feel and move with greater freedom after six weeks of supplementation, and furthermore, continue to improve for many months after, when they continued the omega-6 supplementation.

Therefore, you just increase the intake of omega-3 and omega-6 and glean the benefits. Unfortunately, it is not as easy as it first seems, as the poor dietary and lifestyle choices you make will inhibit the powerful beautifying and disease fighting properties of them. Excess saturated fats, trans fatty acids, sugar intake, smoking, alcohol, and certain illnesses (such as diabetes, cancer, and viral infections) will not allow the body to breakdown and utilise the omega-3 and omega-6 compounds, and therefore, not fully appreciate the benefits. And to make things more interesting, omega-3 in excessive amounts will lower both your 'good' and bad' cholesterol. Therefore, it is important to reduce the barriers and stay within the recommendations of the uptake of omega-3 and omega-6 if you want to look younger and stay healthier for longer.

Monounsaturated fatty acids

Sources: Vegetable and nut oils such as olive, peanut, hazelnut, almond, and avocado and in smaller quantities in nuts and seeds such as, Brazil, cashew, sesame, and pumpkin

Follow the 'mono' way to a healthy heart and learn how and why the people of the Mediterranean have benefited for centuries from reduced heart diseases. Studies have proved that these health benefits have been derived from a high consumption of foods containing monounsaturated fatty acids (such as olives and extra virgin olive oil). These oils are typically high in vitamin E, a powerful anti-oxidant (a substance that protects the body against free radical damage), and with regular use, especially in place of unsaturated and trans fatty acids, people show:

- reduced cholesterol levels
- lower risks of heart disease, diabetes, asthma protection from cancers (such as breast, and colon)

- healthier skin
- a boosted immune system

What is it about olive oil?

A food, which has been around, mostly in the Mediterranean area (until recently) for over six thousand years, and during this time it has been used as a food, medicine, and fuel. The 'magic' of extra virgin olive oil is likely due to the plentiful polyphenols and their antioxidant activity. These are known to have anti-inflammatory, anti-oxidant, and anti-blood thickening actions. As with any potential health food, simply including olive oil to a food plan that is unhealthy will negate any of its potential health benefits.

A study published in the Journal of the American College of Cardiology, looked into the levels of free radicals harmful to cholesterol, which increased after eating. The study showed that when the people in this study ate a breakfast containing extra virgin olive oil, far fewer of these damaging free radicals were present than would normally be seen after a meal. However, when they ate the same breakfast containing olive oil with fewer polyphenols, the beneficial effects were almost non-existent, and had increased the concentrations of cholesterol damaging free radicals.

How do you take your olive oil?

In a recent study by the European Food Research and Technology, it was shown that exposure to heat and light will remove the majority of the 'magic' polyphenols, and their related health benefits, which are found in cold pressed extra virgin oil.

To ensure you receive the maximum benefits from olive oil here are some tips on how to store and purchase it:

- Purchase cold pressed extra virgin oil (a better flavour and holds the most polyphenols)
- Look for dark tinted containers (or ones which do not allow light through)
- Keep olive oil away from direct sunlight or heat
- Store in a cupboard when not in use

Trans-fatty acids

Sources include hundreds of food brands and products such as: Breakfast cereals; cakes, cookies, muffins, pies, donuts; corn chips, potato chips; crackers; French fries; bakery products, toaster pastries, waffles, pancakes; frozen entrees, snack foods, and meals such as meats, fish (such fish sticks), pizza, burritos; instant mashed potatoes; low-fat ice creams; margarines, shortening; noodle soup cups; peanut butter (except fresh-ground); sauce mixes; whipped toppings

Trans unsaturated fatty acids, or trans fats, a brand new entry into the 'fats' list, an artificial product of the 20th century. These trans fats are solid fats produced artificially by heating liquid vegetable oils. This process, partial hydrogenation, causes the trans fat to remain in a solid state at room temperature and has been commercially used since 1909 but with greater frequency since the 1960's, to increase food shelf life, to reduce costs, and ironically, improve taste (making it less oily). This new process also introduced new products to the market, such as, margarine, which was trumpeted, in error, as a new 'health' product as a replacement for butter. Past studies have been confirmed more recently, which strengthen the case against trans fats. They have a negative impact on the blood lipids of a person, which cause increased risks of coronary heart disease, with researchers concluding that removing trans fats from food could prevent tens of thousands of heart attacks and cardiac deaths each year in the United States.

The Food and Drug Administration in the United States, bowing to this kind of evidential pressure, as of January 1, 2006, issued guidelines that ensure trans fat must be listed on food labels. The negative effects to you health of excess consumption trans fats are:

- increased risk of coronary heart disease
- increasing of 'bad' cholesterol
- reductions in 'good' cholesterol

There are no benefits associated with consuming trans fatty acids and they should be severely restricted from any nutritional plan aimed at preserving your health and well-being. Choose to make your own meals and deserts and avoid the prepared and packaged foods found in most supermarkets or fast food outlets such as:

Food product	Trans fat content
French-fries (med)	8g
Potato crisps (small bag)	3g
Doughnut (medium)	5g
Cookies (x3)	2g
A candy / chocolate bar	3g
Slice of cake (80g)	4.5g

Ways to avoid the trans fat trap:

- Read the ingredients list for the 'hidden' trans fats
  - o Partially hydrogenated fat

- o Hydrogenated vegetable oil
  - o Shortening
- Stick to home country products - not all products, especially imported one, have correct labelling
- Replace trans fat and saturated fat with monounsaturated and polyunsaturated fats
- Reduce your intake on fried foods, fast foods, and commercially processed foods
- Beware of products that offer "no cholesterol", "cholesterol free", 'low fat' and such like, because can contain relatively high levels of trans fat

Derived fats: Cholesterol

Sources: Eggs, turkey, chicken, pork, beef, lamb, meat organs (liver, kidney, brains), dairy products (ice cream, milk, cheese, butter), certain fish (shrimps, sardines), cod liver oil

Cholesterol is wholly found in animal products and not available in any plants structures. Cholesterol is the most recognised derived fat, and is an 'add-on' to the fats group; it shares some of the other fat compound physical and chemical characteristics, such as its inability to mix with water; and it is for this reason it can be viewed as a fat. Even if you followed a 'no cholesterol' food plan, your body would produce its own adequate supply to perform the required body functions. It is an important component of many tissues and performs many vital functions, such as, in the production of vitamin D, adrenal gland, and sex hormones. Clusters of cholesterol are carried through the blood stream and these clusters are identified as lipoproteins. The main three types of lipoproteins are the:

1. **High density lipoproteins (HDL)** - 'good' cholesterol
   Function as a 'scavenger' to remove cholesterol from the artery walls. The lower the HDL's the greater the risk of heart disease.
2. **Low density proteins (LDL)** - 'bad' cholesterol
   Cause clogging and plaque formation in the arteries. The higher the LDL's the greater the risk of heart disease.
3. **Very low-density protein (VLDL)** - 'bad' cholesterol
   Degradation of VLDL in the liver will form the 'bad' cholesterol LDL.

Cholesterol measures, such as the LDL count and total cholesterol serum levels, can predict the risks of coronary heart disease. A food intake of excess cholesterol will eventually lead to atherosclerosis, a clogging of the medium and large arteries. In a controlled study, spanning seven and ten years into the relationship between cholesterol levels and heart disease, the results showed that reductions in cholesterol reduced the risks of heart disease. Improvements in the coronary artery risk were shown to be in a ratio of 1:2; for instance, for every 1% reduction in cholesterol levels in was shown to have a 2 % reduction in the risk of heart disease. You should aim to reduce your intake of cholesterol, as is not an essential nutrient and your body can make its own adequate supply. Avoiding foods such as eggs, animal organs, dairy products, and some fish (and oils) and products made from them, will reduce your exposure to excess cholesterol. Here is a list of common food cholesterol:

Food item		Cholesterol (mg)
Chicken and noodles	1 cup	103
Cheesecake	1 piece	170
Duck roasted	½ duck	197
Egg	x 1	210
Butter	½ cup	247
Quiche	1 slice	285
Pizza with cheese	1 slice	56
Double cheese burgers with bacon		145
Large milk shakes		168
Croissant, sausage with egg and cheese		225– 255
Egg muffin		235
Sausage muffins		255
Scrabbled eggs x 2		425

Any surprises? Your body produces all the cholesterol it needs, any additions in the shape of dietary cholesterol will in high quantities increase you risks of heart disease.

The Micronutrients
Vitamins
Vitamins are nutrients you only need in small amounts, which are vital to almost all body functions. You can only obtain them from consuming food or supplements (or a little sunlight in the case of vitamin D). Most of the required vitamins can be supplied by eating a variety of fruits, vegetables, nuts, seeds, and whole grains. You will find a full listing of essential vitamins and their food sources in the appendix at the back of this book; below are some highlighted health benefits:

- Essential for growth and development of a 'new you' everyday
- Prevents premature aging and ensures you look and feel great

- Facilitates maximum energy production and relieves you of toxic elements
- Increases your mental and physical capacities
- Boosts the immune system, protecting you from illness and disease

Vitamins are divided into two categories: fat-soluble and water-soluble. Fat-soluble vitamins are found in fats and oils in foods, and tend to accumulate in the body: vitamin A (and the beta carotene precursor to vitamin A production), D, E, and K. Water-soluble vitamins dissolve in water and mix easily in the blood and are stored long enough for use and then excreted.

All for one and one for all
It is the sum of all the individual components that go into your body, which make it operate to its full capacity, and continually work towards maintaining a healthy balanced body. Vitamins (along with minerals, fibre, carbohydrates, essential amino acids, and fats) should be viewed as a whole package and not as numerous separate entities. It is important not to make one vitamin, more or less important, than the other. It is true that some vitamins are needed in more quantity than others are, but essentially, if any vitamin intake produces either a deficiency or an overdose situation then it is likely to do more harm than good.

Too many supplements
You cannot hope to take a health food supplement and expect to receive the same benefits as you would if you consumed the equivalent food sources, or hope to correct all the made choices made in a unhealthy diet. The supplement industry thrives on people who have cupboards stacked with every available lotion, pill, and potion; for which they need a supplement diary just to keep on top of their daily ritualistic supplementation, with a milligram of this, a milligram of that, a few International units here, or micrograms there. They are sold the false hope that they will receive good health and protection from illness and disease. Any vitamin taking in excess has no extra benefits to your health and will only be excreted from the body, or put more bluntly, just money down the drain. The health supplement industry is a global multi-million one, hitting the billion-pound mark in some countries. It will continue to increase its sales and profits and long as people believe that they are building a protective wall around their good health.

The truth of the matter is that people will only ever be exposed to deficiency cases in only but a few key vitamins, and the message is to those people, as always is, to eat more fruit, vegetables, and whole grains.

Minerals

Like vitamins, minerals perform many essential functions in the body, and reside in various body tissues and fluids. They freely occur in nature and are neither animal nor vegetable; they are inorganic. There are varying amounts in most of the things you eat and a well-balanced food intake, which includes a variety of fruits, vegetables, legumes, and whole grains will easily fulfil your mineral requirements. Here are some of their health benefits (refer to Appendices, for a listing of minerals and sources:

- Essential for strong and healthy body: repairing and the growth of bones, teeth, muscle, connective tissue
- Fundamental in your heart functions and in the production of blood; maintains normal blood pressure
- Ensure you have high energy levels and tension free muscles
- Provide repair and rejuvenation; giving your cells protection against harmful chemical reactions fighting against premature ageing
- A daily detox: effectively removes toxic chemicals
- Maximise your reproductive functions
- Optimises your Resting Metabolic Rate
- Increase your brain functions and abilities to concentrate
- Promotes your mental balance; avoiding irritability, anxiety, and other mentally destabilising conditions
- Provides components for digestion, promoting fat and carbohydrate metabolism

The essential to life minerals, are referred to as **major** minerals and are those requiring a recommended daily allowance of more than 300 milligrams. These are calcium, phosphorus, potassium, sulphur, sodium, and chorine.

The rest are referred to as **minor** minerals with recommended daily allowances of less than 150 milligrams, and trace minerals of less than one milligram. As was the case with vitamins, minerals should be consumed through fresh and seasonal (chemical and pesticide free) fruits, vegetables, nuts, seeds, and whole grains.

Deficiencies in the average person are rare for those following such a food plan, and any over supply of minerals leads to no extra physiological benefits whatsoever. Moreover, excessively high intake of certain minerals can be toxic to the body and have its own health repercussions.

**How to tell if you need to take a supplement or not;
here is a checklist to help decide:**

- Do you eat less than **five** or more servings of fruit and vegetables per day?
- Are there food groups such as meat, fruit, vegetable, or dairy, which you do not eat?
- Do you follow a low calorie or an overly restrictive diet?
- Do you have any diseases of the liver, gallbladder, intestines, or pancreas, or have had surgery on your digestive system?
- Do you smoke?
- Do you drink alcohol in more than the recommended quantities?
- Do you partake in exercise or physical activity where sweat excessively?
- Are you older than sixty?

Three extra questions for women

- Are you a postmenopausal woman?
- Are you a woman who has heavy menstrual bleeding?
- Are you pregnant or trying to get pregnant?

If you answered 'Yes' to **any** of the questions above then you could be in need of an additional vitamin and mineral 'assurance' policy.

The vitamin and mineral assurance policy
Any standard multivitamin available in any retailer, which supplies the recommended daily allowances of the vitamins and minerals, will supply you with more than enough of the few you may or may not be missing. The cost of this insurance policy – an annul expense of around £20-£60. This can be considered a very inexpensive assurance premium considering the potential health benefits perceived. Here is how to make the best choice:

- Always check the label
- Avoid mega doses of any vitamin or mineral and the inadequate ones which have Recommended Daily Allowance of less than 100%
- Choose a one-a-day multi vitamin / mineral product that has the standard 100% Recommended Daily Allowance for all the vitamins and minerals (the exception is Calcium)
- Watch out for the differing qualities of supplies and 'added' ingredients
- If it does not have an expiry date do not purchase it
- Follow the storage instructions on the label

Chapter 8

Healing food

Nourishment for living is the study of the foods you need to consume, in order to ensure your basic life sustaining needs. By understanding nourishment and the intricate role it plays in preventing the manifestation of illness and disease, the more the focus will move away from being reactive to the needs of good health and will look much more closely at a proactive approach. Healing foods are your gateway to a better health and well-being.

As technology improves, scientists have the capability to delve into the body, and observe its functioning in finite detail, and this includes the intricate actions and reactions that take place when we eat food. It will be an enlightening and liberating experience to see within human body cells, as it will produce a revolutionary new understanding into why certain foods can lead to decreased energy, premature ageing, illness, and disease; it will be observed and unfold like a space-age home movie.

Before you can fully appreciate the importance of nourishment and your future health, it is wise to take a brief look back at what has occurred in the previous years and how it has shaped the current situation. It will reveal great insights into the problems of the 21st century people and lay down a blueprint of how you should approach your nourishment from this day forward.

From 40,000BC onwards, the first human representations were believed to be hunter-gatherers and their lives revolved around their procurement of food to survive. Their food intake, which has been revealed by the evidence-based examination of their bones and teeth, consisted of wild plants, fruits, vegetables, and a low amount of food from animal origin. They adapted to their surroundings and created crude tools to gather foods from trees, the soil, and to hunt and scavenge.

Environmental conditions and seasonal variations dictated food choices, where the ability to store non-perishable foods such as; nuts, bulbs, fruits, and root vegetables became necessities to survive through the seasons. Clothing and fire provided the means to make the next step, such as surviving harsh winters, living in enclosed spaces, and in the search to process and find new foods. There is evidence that around 10,000BC simple food processes had been introduced such as, the pounding, grinding, scraping, roasting, and baking; this allowed the use of wild grains and pulses.

The last Ice Age was survived and those peoples began to prosper in an environment where wild grasses, cereals, and legumes flourished and animals such as, sheep, goats, cattle, and pigs were being domesticated. Where the earlier ancestors probably derived two-thirds of their food intake from fruits, vegetables, and nuts, the onset of agriculture saw this figure decrease substantially with a subsequent decrease in meat consumption.

These initial steps of humans formed the basis of the food nutrients required by the body, with which the people of today use to live a healthy balanced life. Survival instincts have drawn the lines for the blueprint of nutrients, which are common knowledge to people today: carbohydrates, fibre, proteins, fats, vitamins, and minerals, giving you many opportunities to meet the nutritional needs of your body.

The machines arrived
Subtle changes over tens of thousands of years brought humans to a situation where they no longer led nomadic lifestyles. The gathering of people around sources of water and fertile soils created villages and towns, and a climate where culture and knowledge prospered. Populations thrived on reliable food sources, which allowed for food surpluses and wider ranges of foods available for storage. People thrived on these new riches, and populations increased rapidly and the first signs of cities appeared. The industrial revolution changed everything.

The 20th century saw the change from manual and animal powered agriculture to a motorised one, from a nomadic lifestyle to a settled one. The competition was on, to produce more and more, bigger and better; specialised selection processes searched for the highest yielding crops and animal produce least affected by disease. Simultaneously, chemical fertilisers, insecticides, new feeding practices, and constantly improving agriculture tools and machines, and relatively new strides in food science introduced more and more produce to the market. Improving transport infrastructure such as the road, rail, sea, and air networks delivered the increased quantities of foods faster and further distances. All people had to do now, was eat it.

A relatively few number of decades had brought with it quantitative and qualitative food and nutrient combinations, which had not previously been encountered over the entire period of human evolution. Humans are the only living species that have strayed so far from its evolutionary blueprint. They boast high consumptions of foods with ingredients such as, excess salt, sugar (and all its guises: brown sugar, raw sugar, corn syrup, corn-syrup solids, high-fructose corn syrup, malt syrup, maple syrup, pancake syrup, fructose sweetener, liquid fructose, honey, molasses, anhydrous dextrose, and crystal dextrose), refined flours, and extraordinary amounts of trans fatty acids. With all the adaptations mentioned, one thing is constant; you are left with foods with fewer nutrients and increased calorific impacts. By eating more processed foods, you will increase calorie intake, but receive in return, fewer essential nutrients. Therefore, you have to eat more to supply the shortfall in essential nutrients, which opens the door on a wealth of modern epidemics such as, obesity (though not a modern disease, it has reached worrying proportions in the last thirty years), diabetes, heart disease, hypertension, and cancer, and many other illnesses.

A 100-year-old menace
Though you can be forgiven for thinking that the role of poor nutrition and its related diseases such as obesity is a new phenomenon, it is not. As far back as the 15th November 1885 an article was written in The Washington Post titled 'How to Cure Obesity'. In 1943, Dr Quigley published a book called 'The Modern Malnutrition' and in his introduction talks at length at the increase of 'bad' foods such as white flour, sugar, canned and packaged foods, cold storage meats; at the expense of 'good' natural foods such as fruits, whole grains, and vegetables. He goes on to say that, 'The selling of bad food has become one of the biggest if not actually the biggest of business enterprises....The bad qualities of certain foods were admitted. It was conceded that white flour and sugar were producers of the most dangerous diseases.'

In 1939, with an expert view of the Industrial Age and the changes happening to the food industry, Jean Bogert, a nutritionist, reflected on the growing promotion and use of refined cereal grains, processed foods, and sugar at the expense of fruit and vegetables. 'The machine age has had the effect of forcing upon the peoples of the industrial nations the most gigantic human feeding experiment ever attempted.'

In a recent study, published in the American Journal of Clinical Nutrition, it was shown that people in the United States receive over 72% of their calories from dairy products, cereals, refined sugars, refined vegetable oils, and alcohol. These items or their processed offspring such as, cookies, cakes, bakery foods, breakfast cereals, bagels, rolls, muffins, crackers, chips, snack foods, pizza, soft drinks, candy, ice cream, condiments, and salad dressings, were just not available as options pre-agricultural revolution.

Humans have a similar genetic make up as they did 40,000 years ago, and the blueprint laid down by a long line of ancestors should continue be the basis for your daily food intakes and continued prosperity. Survival instincts mapped the blueprint in 40,000 years and now humans are faced with commercial instincts wiping them out in just over a hundred. The relatively split-second evolutionary time change in dietary habits has reduced the body's ability to adapt quick enough to these changes, and the consequences of which are causing illness, diseases, premature deaths, and major concerns for the future of human health and quality of life.

Industrial Age diseases

Millions of people have been affected by these rapid changes in nutritional content. In the last three decades alone, a saturation point has been reached in the communications received from media and government backed organisations. Although the 'health' messages have their foundations laid in sand, and susceptible to change at any moment, they are to be commended, as the aim is a healthier population.

Yet in this same period the cases of heart disease, stroke, type 2 diabetes, cancer, and obesity, coined the 'diseases of affluence' have grown to become major epidemics. The change in diets over the last hundred years or so have accelerated the prevalence of these diseases, and with the advances in food science and technology there is growing evidence that new detrimental factors have been and continue to be introduced to a person's food diet. Not only has the diseases of affluence grown in this time but relatively new problems have also seen growth, such as, Alzheimer's disease, osteoporosis, senile dementia, and depression.

Ruled by your heart

The British Heart Foundation's recent figures for heart and circulatory diseases show that coronary heart disease and strokes, now kills over 230,000 people; that is more than one in three of all deaths that occur in the United Kingdom. Furthermore, there are more than 1.2 million people living in the United Kingdom who have had a heart attack and over 66% of people have cholesterol levels in excess of government guideline targets. Although the populations differ vastly, around 70 million in the United Kingdom compared to close to 280 million in the United States, the cardiovascular death rate percentages are almost identical, at around 40% of all deaths in the respective countries.

More than 70 million Americans have one or more types of cardiovascular disease, which also represents the leading cause of mortality in the United States. About 90% of middle-aged Americans will develop high blood pressure in their lifetime, and nearly 70% of those who have it now do not have it under control. The cost in Europe for cardiovascular and coronary heart disease is over €200 billion per year. While in the United States, the 2005 health costs of heart disease and stroke is projected to exceed $394 billion.

Diabetes – a silent disease
People with diabetes have a shortage of insulin or a decreased ability to use it. Uncontrolled diabetes will cause glucose and fats to remain in the blood, and over time, vital organs are damaged, eventually causing illness and disease such as, heart disease, stroke, blindness, kidney failure, limb amputations, and flu and pneumonia.

In the last fifteen years, this disease has been diagnosed at alarming rates. The World Health Organisation estimate the current number of diabetes suffers at 170 million and predict a number closer to 300 million in less than ten years time. The United Kingdom reports over two million with diabetes attributing over 7,000 deaths per year to it, and the United States has seen the people diagnosed with diabetes double since 1990 to 14.6 million (2005). The cost to the United States alone was estimated in 2002 at $132 billion. Moreover, the silent disease has tens of millions who people who live with elevated levels of blood sugar, and are in line to develop full-blown diabetes, but are unaware of it.

Counting the costs of cancer
Cancer has no boundaries or borders and affects people regardless of location, status, wealth, age, or gender, contributing to seven million deaths per year. It can attack and spread within any tissue in the body and the most common worldwide are lung and stomach for men, and breast and cervical cancer for women. The World Health Organisation reports that over eleven million people are diagnosed with cancer every year. Moreover, they predict that an additional sixteen million new cases will be reported every year by 2020.

The health care costs and loss of productivity runs into hundreds of billions of dollars, with the United States contributing over $210 billion alone. China has 20% of the world's total of new cancer cases at over two million, with North America accounting for close to 15%. In the United States, cancer claims over half a million deaths per year and reports over a million new cases in the same period, making it the second leading cause of deaths in the country. More than two people in every thousand will perish because of cancer in the United Kingdom.

An obese issue

According to the World Health Organisation, in excess of one billion people are overweight with 30% of them clinically obese. Developed and developing countries have seen increasing rates of obesity coupled with an increase of chronic diseases such as, type 2 diabetes, cardiovascular disease, hypertension and stroke, and certain forms of cancer. The burden of obesity has been attributed to factors such as subsidized agriculture and multi-national companies providing cheap unhealthy foods, and modernisation that promotes inactivity. More than 50% of adults in western populations are overweight or obese. In the United States, data published in the 2003-2004 National Health and Nutrition Examination Survey shows that 66% of the population is overweight with the obesity rate at 32%. In European countries people who are overweight or obese is likely to top 150 million by 2010.

Urban areas of many developing countries are the first to show an increase in overweight and obesity. In China, the rural areas report obesity rates of less than 5%, whereas in the new rapidly expanding cities the obesity rates are closer to 20%. While it is likely that developed countries will see a slowing down in any major yearly increases, the growth is likely to come from the developing countries as they play 'catch-up'.

Bones of contention

It was not until 1994 when the World Health Organization identified Osteoporosis as a priority health issue. Osteoporosis is reported to affect an estimated 75 million people in Europe, USA, and Japan, with a third of women and a fifth of men suffering from some kind of bone damage.

Osteoporosis is a disease in which the density and quality of bone are reduced, leading to weakness and increased risk of bone fractures. It is a global problem, which is increasing in significance as the population of the world expands, ages, is physically inactive, and lacks the adequate supplies of vitamin and minerals. The costs to national healthcare systems from osteoporosis-related hospitalisation are staggering; in the United States, the annual direct medical costs, not including any economic related costs, runs at over $20 billion. In Europe, for every one thousand osteoporosis attributed fractures it is estimated that the direct healthcare costs are €3.7 million.

Health is wealth; looking after your cell bank

The trillions of cells, which make up your body are the fundamental elements of life and are the smallest 'living' organisms in the body. They operate on the nutrients you supply and this allows them to function efficiently. Repairing and growing where required, communicating and responding to the signals from the body senses and environment. A lack of nutrients will diminish the body functions, and subsequent exposure to environmental toxins can cause damage to your cells' DNA, and can result in illness and disease. This mutated cell DNA can reduce your ability to produce energy and lead to pain, inflammation, and tumours.

Eating to vitality
By understanding how food and nutrients affect the health of your cells, you not only know what foods are beneficial, but how and why a food plan that features nutrient-rich, toxic chemical and additive free whole foods can promote your optimal health. To make things easier, below are the most advantageous healing and energising foods:

MaxLife70 healing and energising foods

MaxLife21 vegetables
Asparagus; Aubergine (eggplant); Beetroot; Bell peppers; **Broccoli** *; Brussels sprouts; Cabbage; **Carrots** *; Cauliflower; Celery; Cucumber Green beans: runner beans & broad beans; Green peas; Kale; Mushroom; Okra (ladies fingers); Spinach ; Sweet potato; Tomato; Turnip Greens

MaxLife21 fruits
Apple*; Apricot; Banana; Berries (such as blueberries, cranberries, raspberries, and strawberries); Cherries; Citrus fruits (such as lemon, lime, orange, nectarine, and grapefruit); Fig (fresh); Grapes; **Olives***; Pear; Peach; Plum; Pomegranate; Watermelon

MaxLife7 Beans & Legumes
Kidney beans; Lima beans; Pinto beans, Black-eyed beans, and **soybeans***; Chickpeas (garbanzo); Lentils (red, yellow, green)

MaxLife7 Nuts, Seeds, & Oil
Almonds*; Flaxseeds; Hazelnut; Olive oil; Sesame seeds; Sunflower seeds; Pumpkin seeds

MaxLife7 Whole Grains
Barley; Bran; Buckwheat; **Whole oats***; Rice (wild brown); Rye; Whole wheat

MaxLife7 Fresh Herbs
Basil; Coriander; Parsley; Peppermint leaves; Rosemary; Sage; Thyme

The MaxLife7 SUPER Foods *

These seven super foods deserve an extra mention and each has their own powers to take you the extra step to improving health: broccoli, carrots, apples, olives, soybeans, almonds, and oats.

SUPER Food 1:   Broccoli

It started life back in Italy, hence its Italian derived name from 'broccolo' meaning cabbage sprout. As the name suggests it is a part of the cabbage family and a close relative of the cauliflower. In half a cup of broccoli, you get the recommended daily intake of vitamin C and K, followed by excellent supplies of vitamin A, folate, and dietary fibre. The researchers suggest that broccoli stands florets and stalks above any of the other vegetables, for many good reasons; here are a few of them:

- **Cancer Protection** - The elements in broccoli boost the body's protective capabilities and act as a 'sweeper' clearing out potentially dangerous cancer causing substances.

- **Repairs sun-damaged skin** - A little sun is good for you, and a great source of vitamin D. However, too much exposure can lead to damage of the skin and the potential to develop skin cancer. Broccoli in a coordinated effort between its own elements and the body's enzymes has the fantastic ability to repair the damage caused by sun exposure to your skin. So a little sunshine and a cup of broccoli will allow you the benefits gained in the sun and ensure you do not increase your risk of skin cancer.

- **Protects from heart disease** - It has been proven to produce a significant reduction in heart disease risk. The study published in the European Journal of Clinical Nutrition concluded that those who have diets rich in flavonoids, found in broccoli and apples, had gained 20% reductions in their heart disease risk.

- **Stronger Bones** - Broccoli is rich in the components, which help keep your bones strong; it supplies 62 milligrams of vitamin C and 37 milligrams of calcium, in half a cup. It supplies both the most abundant mineral found in your bones (and body), and the vitamin best suited to transport it there, all in half a cup. No other fruit, vegetable or dairy product can offer this wealthy combination.

- **Prevents ulcers** - Rich in sulforaphane, broccoli has the ability to prevent, and may even offer a treatment against, the ulcer-causing bacteria *Helicobacter pylori*.

SUPER Food 2:   **Carrots**

The carrot is believed to have originated in the Middle East regions where its health benefits were widely utilised. Its name comes from the Latin word 'carota'. Just one carrot is enough to supply you with your daily requirement of vitamin A (and its precursors the 'carotenes'), and K. It also has a healthy supply of vitamin C, dietary fibre, and potassium. The Chinese have for thousands of years prescribed this root vegetable as a way to boost your internal organ functions, give you energy, and used it as an antiseptic. Researchers in the east and west have confirmed its healing and preventative qualities with studies, which show the carrot provides protection against some cancers and heart disease. In addition, they will not only look after your insides by cleansing the damaging free radicals, but also take care of the outside to, by encouraging healthy skin, hair, bones, and eyesight.

- **Carotenoids fight heart disease** - A study carried out with older adults showed that daily consumption of a carotene-packed carrot reduced their risk of heart disease by up to 60%, compared to those who ate less.

- **Reduce your cancer risks** - Carrots are the richest source of carotenoids, and just half a cup gives you your recommended allowance. A high carotenoids intake has been shown in various studies to reduce the risk of cancer, such as, lung, breast, colon, gastric, bladder, and prostrate. Just one-a-day and you can cut your risks of lung cancer by 50%. Trials in China reported a statistically significant reduction of cancer mortality rate after supplementation with beta-carotene, vitamin E, and selenium. Furthermore, a study published in the Journal of Agricultural and Food Chemistry showed that falcarinol, an element naturally found in carrots, was shown in experiments to prevent the growth and spread of cancerous lesions, and their progress to tumours.

- **Improved vision** - The carotenoid, beta-carotene helps to protect vision, especially night vision, and in older adults, helps prevent cataracts the leading cause of blindness.

SUPER Food 3:   **Apples**

The 'pome' fruit or apple in Latin has come a long way since its origins in Europe and Asia, and can now boast several thousand different varieties and a worldwide availability. Its mix of fructose, fibre, flavonoids, vitamin C and K, deliver health in every mouthful. 'An apple a day will keep the doctor away', is a proverb recounted for hundreds of years pointing to the health benefits of the apple. Known more as an old wives tale then, it has now been fully vindicated in recent years by the hundreds of subsequent studies, which have confirmed that apples have a role to play in reducing the risk of various diseases, such as cancer, heart disease, asthma, and type 2 diabetes. Add to this apples ability to increase lung function and help you lose weight, the apple is truly a Super Food!

- **Reduce your lung cancer risks** - Apples are one of the fruits that have been frequently linked in studies to lung cancer and its risks. In these studies, it was shown that just one apple a day was enough to reduce your risks of lung cancer. Furthermore, in a case control study published in the Journal of the National Cancer Institute, there was a 40 to 50% decreased risk in lung cancer in participants with the highest intake of flavonoids, in comparison to the people with lower intakes. It also prevents the further growth of cancer. In a study looking at colon cancer, apples proved to be a potent force against the spreading activity of cancer, and it was the phytochemicals in apples, which were shown to be responsible for inhibiting the growth of the tumour cells.

- **Banish the 'bad' cholesterol** - Reduce the 'bad' cholesterol in you liver and plasma, and lower the triglyceride levels. The combination of fibre and the active elements of the apple support the disease-fighting function. The study proved that it is better to eat the apple whole in order to extract the maximum reductions in cardiovascular disease risks, when compared to its juice or dietary supplements.

- **Heart disease risks reduced** - In a study of 40,000 people, which had a nine-year follow-up review, it showed that participants who consumed apples were associated with reduced risks of cardiovascular disease. The Women's Health Study looked at the relationship between the disease-fighting flavonoids in the apples and the risks of cardiovascular disease and showed that the people who consumed the most flavonoids had a 35% reduction in the risk of cardiovascular episodes.

- **Improve your lung function and reduce risks of asthma** - Reduce the incidence of asthma and improve your lung function, on your way to better health by eating apples. In a Finnish study involving 10,000 men and women, it was shown that the flavonoids in apples were associated with a lower risk of asthma. Moreover, a study of over 13,000 adults in the Netherlands, reported that apple intake was positively associated with pulmonary function and negatively associated with chronic obstructive pulmonary disease.

- **Diabetes risks reduced** - In the same Finnish study involving 10,000 adults, the consumption of apples reduced risks of type 2 diabetes. The peel of an apple has a major concentration of quercetin, and this has been associated with type 2 diabetes risk reductions.

- **Losing weight with apples** - In a randomised study of 400 adults in Brazil, after being split into three groups, were observed for 12 weeks while their food intakes were supplemented by an apple, a pear, or an oat cookie. It was shown that participants in the group who were supplemented with a fruit had lost on average 1.21kg at the end of the study (the oat cookie group experienced no significant weight loss). Furthermore, the fruits also significantly reduced the blood sugar levels when compared to those who ate the oat cookies.

SUPER Food 4:   Olives

One of the oldest known foods to humans, with its origins planted in the Mediterranean countries and islands. The olive is looked on as a symbol of peace and wisdom, with mentions in the Qur'an, the Bible, and Egyptian and Greek mythologies. Past generations used the olive tree to provide food, fuel, wood, medicine, and even used it to ward off evil spirits by burning the dried leaves of the tree. Olives are a very good source of monounsaturated fats and a good source of vitamin E, dietary fibre, and the minerals: sodium, iron, copper, and the phytonutrient compound polyphenols and flavonoids. This combination protects your body cells, organs, and the energy producing 'machines' mitochondria. Olives have significant health benefits and they have been found to:

- **Reduce inflammation** - Olives have been shown to reduce inflammation and the severity of conditions such as asthma and arthritis. It helps by reducing the high levels of internal cell damage, which are thought to cause these debilitating diseases.
- **Protects the basics of life** - It goes after and directly neutralizes free radicals and fights the DNA damage that may eventually reappear as mutated or cancerous cells. Protection is also offered to cellular processes such as energy production, ensuring optimum performance. A study published in the Journal of Medicine and Food showed that even olive tree leaf extract has the ability to fight the damages of internal body stresses.
- **Provides you with a potent anti-cancer weapon** – A recent study provided research, which showed that olive derived elements were a non-toxic powerful antioxidant and a potent anti-cancer compound, which directly disrupted the proliferation and migration of cancer tumour cells of the colon.
- **Reduce your risk of heart disease** - One of the latest studies conducted into the health benefits of the olive, proved that 'oleuropein' an olive constituent, was proven to reduce total cholesterol and fat concentrations in three and six-week controlled

studies. The research paper concluded that not only were the risks of heart disease reduced, but that it also offered the possibility of its use as a treatment for those suffering from the disease.

SUPER Food 5:   **Soy beans**

The soybean is a species of legume, a relation of the clover and pea, and a native to eastern Asia. In just one cup of cooked soybeans, there is more than 50% of your recommended daily protein requirement; this high quality protein has a complete supply of the essential amino acids and other equally beneficial phytonutrients vital for good health. Look to avoid processed, purified, and genetically modified versions of soy products, and choose the minimally processed foods such as, whole soybeans and flour, tofu, and tempeh. These type products will supply the optimum amounts available of the numerous minerals, dietary fibre, and omega-3 fatty acids to be found in them, and in doing so offers the maximum available health benefits such as:

- **Reduced risks of coronary artery disease** - In a study published in the American Journal of Clinical Nutrition, soybeans were proven to reduce 'bad' cholesterol and triglycerides (the basic units of fat), while increasing the levels of the 'good' cholesterols. The combined effect of all three actions is the reduced risks of coronary artery disease. The isoflavones (a phytonutrient) found in soy beans also seem to improve the health of your coronary arteries and may even lower your blood pressure. The essential fatty acids alpha-linolenic and omega-3 have already been established as having coronary benefits. This was further confirmed, when in a study involving close to 65,000 women, soy products were associated with multiple coronary benefits, such as an 86% reduction in non-fatal myocardial infarction.

- **Fewer and smaller fat cells** – If you cannot reduce the fat around your waist then eating soybeans may have an answer. A study published in the journal Endocrinology suggests active compounds found in soy may help you stay lean, by causing you to produce fewer and smaller fat cells.

- **Super strong bones** - The results of numerous studies indicate that there is a beneficial combination between isoflavones found in soy compounds and the body's estrogenic compounds. This synergy results in an increase in the body's own estrogen and therefore, an increase in bone density essential for strong healthy bones.

- **Diabetes controller** - The excellent source of protein that is found in soybeans is perfect for those who are diabetic and have issue with other sources of protein. The protein-fibre double act helps to control blood sugar levels and gives diabetes patients another weapon in the fight for an improved quality of life.

- **Cancer combatant** – Soy protein and its protective compounds can offer you protection against different types of cancer. A study published in the Journal of Nutrition showed that soy protein may prevent colon cancer and reduce the size and number of tumours that do occur.

- **Master the menopause** - With the consumption of soybeans you can look to eliminate some of the uncomfortable symptoms related to the menopause. The soybeans provide estrogen like compounds and can help replace the reduction of estrogen, and in turn reduce episodes such as hot flushes, in the process.

> **A word of caution**
> People with already existing and untreated thyroid problems, on special calcium prescriptions, and those susceptible to food allergies may seek to use soybeans with caution, upon further advice.

SUPER Food 6:   Almonds

The almond tree was originally located in the Mediterranean region, has now found life in places as far a field as California (which now boasts a thriving almond industry). It is a truly beautiful sight in springtime to see the whitish-pink blossoms make their appearance, and be afforded a clue as to the healthy treasures they hide. The almond is the 'king' of the nuts, though technically it is the seed of a fruit. It is superior in overall performance when compared to the Brazil nut, cashew, hazelnut, macadamia, pecan, pistachio, and the walnut. Boasting higher amounts of protein (one ounce having almost as much as red meat!), dietary fibre, calcium, vitamins E, and B_2 (riboflavin). It is a great source of dietary fat, with nearly 70% of it being monounsaturated; it also has the lowest saturated fat content of all nuts. In addition, it is close to the top of the class of micronutrient content such as iron, zinc, potassium, phosphorus, and magnesium. A handful of almonds will offer great health benefits such as:

- **Eating to stay slim** - A study published in the International Journal of Obesity and Related Metabolic Disorders, showed that a diet enriched with almonds and its high monounsaturated content, was more effective than a diet high in complex carbohydrates. Those on the almond enriched diet consumed 39% of their total calories from fat (25% being monounsaturated) and those on the complex carbohydrate diet only consumed 18% of their total daily calories from fat (5% coming from monounsaturated fat). Both groups were given the same daily calorie intakes with similar protein amounts and after six months, the results were reported: those on the almond enriched diet showed between 50 to 60% greater reductions in their weight / body mass index, waist circumference, and body fat compared to those on the low calorie high carbohydrate diet.

- **Disturbs 'bad' cholesterol production** - Almonds are a source of healthful cell protectors. Research has revealed nine phenolic compounds in almonds, of which eight exhibit strong cell protection activity. The almond, its skin, and the phenolic compounds are well absorbed into the body and are powerfully active in preventing the oxidation of 'bad' cholesterol, the chief culprit of increased heart disease risks.

- **Reduces the 'bad' and improves the 'good'** - In a review of seven clinical studies it was found that by eating just one ounce of almonds daily, as part of a healthy lifestyle, lowered 'bad' cholesterol. The review went on to show that not only did almonds significantly reduce the 'bad' and total cholesterol by 6% and 4% respectively, but also increased the 'good' cholesterol by 6%. This cholesterol-lowering and heart disease risk reducing effect is similar to that of heart-healthy foods such as oats and soy.

- **Diabetes control** - An enriched almond diet, which contained higher levels of monounsaturated fat and protein than one compared to the American Heart Association diet, was shown to reduce the body weight of the participants, and improved the Glycemic control in those with type 2 diabetes.

- **A healthy brain** - Increasing dietary intake of polyunsaturated fatty acids, particularly omega-3, is linked to reduced risk for Alzheimer's disease. Researchers at the University of Illinois, Chicago, showed that the substance, cholinesterase found in almonds, acted like the drug inhibitors used to treat Alzheimer's disease and that the almond enriched diet also reduced the number of Alzheimer deposits.

- **Cancer combative** - With on-going research, the almond is being associated with an important role to play in cancer prevention. The cell protecting polyphenols, vitamin E and dietary fibre in almonds may be the components that exert the greatest cancer preventative effects. In a study published in Cancer Letters the almond enriched diet was shown to activate five anti-proliferative genes compared to the control diets, and the researchers concluded that the increase in anti-proliferation might account for almonds preventative effect on colon cancer.

SUPER Food 7:   Whole oats

Whole oats play an essential role in promoting your overall good health; originating in Asia as wild oats, they have become commonplace in the lives of many. Aside from fibre and protein, whole grain oats can also provide you with a number of essential vitamins and nutrients, including manganese, magnesium, selenium, vitamin B_1 (thiamine), and phosphorus. Eating the recommended servings of whole grain oats each day can also help reduce your chances of developing several serious diseases, such as heart disease, and can help with maintaining a healthier bodyweight.

- **Lowers the risks of developing heart disease** - Whole grain oats are low in saturated fat and cholesterol, and may reduce the risks of heart disease. In research published in the Archives of Internal Medicine, it was shown that eating high fibre foods such as whole grain oats help to prevent heart disease. Close to 10,000 people over a 19 year duration, participated in this study and the people eating the most fibre (21 grams per day) all showed reductions in coronary heart and cardiovascular disease.

- **Maintains ideal bodyweight** - Whole grain oats promote satiety, which is important for weight management, they are high in complex carbohydrates and fibre, and they promote a feeling of fullness. The whole oat is a great food to consume as part of you healthy lifestyle while looking after your weight the natural way.

- **Oats for breakfast** - Eating oats at breakfast has a lower impact on your blood sugar levels when compared to some cereals and bread. More importantly, the effect of an oats based breakfast is a lasting one, which allows people with type 2 diabetes to control their blood sugar levels with greater ease for the rest of the day.

- **Disposing of toxic waste** - Promoting a healthy digestive system, eating oats can ensure the daily removal of toxic waste build-ups within the body. Oats are a good supply of fibre, and this fibre works as a 'magic sponge' mopping up all the disease-causing elements on its way through your digestive system. The compounds in oats also deter infection, by removing their causes and in doing so proceeds to enhance your immune system.

- **Reduces your risk of developing several types of cancer** - The substances in whole grains that help protect against heart disease may also help prevent certain kinds of cancer, including cancers of the colon, stomach, and prostate. Research published by the American Institute for Cancer Research has shown that populations eating diets high in fibre-rich whole grains such as oats have consistently shown lower risks for colon cancer. The outer layer of whole grain oats is the key to reducing your risks, as it is this outer layer, which contains high amounts of phytochemicals, the cancer-fighting substance. It is essential, therefore, you seek to consume whole grain oats as oppose to any commercially refined grains in order to retain the maximum health benefits.

- **Blood pressure moderator** - The DASH diet (Dietary Approaches to Stop Hypertension) is a dietary pattern recommended by health professionals to help promote healthy blood pressure. The diet recommends plenty of whole grains such as oats. Research shows that these whole grains in the DASH diet make important contributions to the overall nutrient intake, as well as, specific nutrients associated with their positive effects on blood pressure.

Use the Food Intake Guidelines that appear in Chapter 10 – Food for thought, to maximise the power of the MaxLife foods and Super foods.

Chapter 9

Venomous food

Food safety is a growing concern; and has been highlighted by several major incidents involving salmonella, E. coli, mad cow disease. Foodborne diseases are usually either infectious or toxic in nature, and are caused by agents that enter the body through the ingestion of food. Every person is at risk of foodborne illnesses and diseases. They are an increasing worldwide burden and estimated figures point to rapid rises in their prevalence in more recent years; there are estimated in excess of 76 million cases reported in the United States, over five million in Australia, and over a million in England. The illness symptoms can include diarrhoea and vomiting, and in long-term infections and severe cases result in death.

Safe food, from farm to fork, is a priority considering the important role it plays in your health and well-being. The responsibility of safe food can be distributed between producers, processors, distributors, retailers, and finally, the consumer. Most consumer concerns can be summed up as:

- Safe food handling: cleanliness, and preparation
- Freshness concerns
- Farming issues
  - o Animal welfare and disease
  - o Pesticides and insecticides
- Food additives and preservatives

New and re-emerging hazards
For the average consumer, 'Freshness' and 'Safe food handling' are considered to be the number one issues regarding food safety. However, in a recent review, 'The global diet: trade and novel infections', it was

shown that the growing and diversifying demands of the global consumer are stretching the food production and distribution practices in order to keep pace. This rapidly evolving production and practices may also be contributing new pathogens and creating 'new' versions of existing compounds. The following is a Top 10 list of the new or re-emerging food hazards you should be aware of and proactively trying to avoid:

The Top 10 - Poisons on a plate

1. Viral additives - *New Entry -*
On Friday, August 18, 2006, the United States Food and Drug Administration approved a 'viral cocktail' for the use on food supplies. This viral cocktail will be sprayed onto foods to tackle the growing problem of antibiotic resistant germs. A Listeria bacterium, for example, has hundreds of different strains and the idea is that these bioengineered viral cocktails (as one virus is not sufficient to remove all strains) will be sprayed onto foods to seek and destroy all of them. When the viral cocktail is sprayed onto food, it seeks out the bacteria and attaches itself to it. This is the start of the end for the bacteria, as the viral cocktail injects its own DNA into it and using the bacteria as food, multiplies inside it. The bacterium tries to defend itself by releasing its own defence mechanism - little poisons called 'endotoxins'. The viral cocktail is too powerful for the bacteria, which explodes leaving both the endotoxins and the viral cocktail in the food and on its way to your local store.

In a recent study published by the American Society for Microbiology, endotoxins (the poisons released by the bacteria) induced in participants a rapid physiological response such as fever, irregular heart patterns, and blood pressure changes. Moreover, other studies have been associated with cancers. How long will it be before the bacterium, which the viral cocktail has been sent to seek and destroy develops a resistance strain to it, possibly turning the bacteria into a killer, in the same way Cholera occurred. The viral cocktail may attack the healthy bacteria you have in your digestive systems or mutate and create new harmful forms of itself within your body. This is of much concern to many people, and should be for you to.

The company that manufactures the viral cocktail Intralytix has already licensed their newly approved viral spray to a multi-national company for use around the world. However, they declined to say which company!

2. Foodborne bacterial and viral infections
Bacteria that cause foodborne illness either by infecting the intestinal tissues directly, or by producing bacterial toxins include pathogens such as Campylobacter jejuni, Salmonella, E. coli, and Listeria

monocytogenes. Salmonellosis is caused by strains of salmonella that are one of the most common and widely distributed foodborne bacterial infections. Millions of human cases are reported worldwide every year and the disease results in thousands of deaths. The World Health Organisation claim there are over 2,500 known strains of salmonella. Since the beginning of the 1990's, strains of Salmonella have begun to demonstrate resistance to a range of single and multi drug treatments available, and are threatening a serious public health problem. In 2005, a study published for Euro Surveillance, highlighted new strains of multi-resistant salmonella in a national outbreak.

In the United States, it is estimated that there are up to four million reported cases per year of salmonellosis. The infection is characterised by symptoms such as, fever, abdominal pain, diarrhoea, nausea, vomiting, and dehydration. The foods that are most commonly associated with bacterial infections are raw meats, poultry, eggs, milk, and dairy products, fish, shrimp, yeast, coconut, sauces and salad dressing, cake mixes, cream-filled desserts and toppings, peanut butter, cocoa, and chocolate. The greatest risk of foodborne illness occurs from catering operations preparing ready to eat foods.

Foodborne viral infections are caused mainly by two types of virus, Norwalk-like viruses, which cause gastroenteritis, and Hepatitis A virus, which causes hepatitis. Norwalk-like viruses cause illnesses that are usually sudden in onset, and are characterized by vomiting, diarrhoea, and abdominal pain. Very few virus particles are needed to cause illness, and so the attack rate in an outbreak can be very high, with the majority of people who ate the contaminated food becoming ill. Because the viruses multiply in the gut, a very large number of virus particles are excreted during the illness. Because of the uncontrollable nature of the symptoms, food can easily become contaminated by infected food handlers, with secondary person-to-person spread being common.

Viral hepatitis has a long incubation period of three to six weeks, with symptoms developing gradually. Symptoms include loss of appetite, malaise, fever, and vomiting, followed by jaundice. Illness usually lasts a few weeks but can last several months, and is usually more severe in adults than in children. The elderly are at particular risk and severe cases can cause death.

3. Chemical residues

This category includes pesticides, biotechnology used in animal agriculture, and industrial chemicals appearing as chronic or sporadic environmental pollutants. Pesticides include insecticides, rodenticides, herbicides, fungicides, and antimicrobials; and it is common for combinations of them to be used on the same crop.

In a recent investigation by the United States Food and Drug Administration, searching for pesticide chemical residues, collected and analysed 2,344 food samples from 43 states, and 4,890 imported samples from 99 countries. Pesticide residue was found in 37.3% of the domestic food samples and 28.2% in the imported ones; and more importantly, pesticide residues, which violated the set tolerances of the Environmental Protection Agency, were found in 2.4% and 6.1% of the domestic and imported food samples respectively. There were 73 pesticides found in wide ranging foods from grains to rice, and pears to strawberries. By their very nature, most pesticides create some risk of harm. Pesticides, dependant on toxicity and exposure, can cause serious harm to humans, animals, or the environment because they are designed to kill or adversely affect living organisms. Pesticides such as organophosphates and carbamates, affect the nervous system, whereas others can cause eye and skin irritations, hormonal and nervous system dysfunction, neurological damage, and some cancers.

All of these common household products are considered pesticides: cockroach sprays, insect repellents for personal use, rat and other rodent poisons, flea and tick sprays, powders, and pet collars, kitchen, laundry, and bath disinfectants, some lawn and garden products, such as weed killers.

In a recent review, 'A Case for Revisiting the Safety of Pesticides: A Closer Look at Neurodevelopment', published in the Environmental Health Perspectives, the head of the review, Colborn argues that there is unequivocal evidence that the exposure of pesticides effects human neurodevelopment. He further added that, government agencies such as the U.S. Environmental Protection Agency's (EPA), should take 'an entirely new approach to determine the safety of pesticides …. It is evident that contemporary acute and chronic toxicity studies are not protective of future generations. The range of doses used in future studies must be more realistic, based on levels found in the environment and human tissue… It is fairly safe to say that every child conceived today in the Northern hemisphere is exposed to pesticides.'

4. Dioxins, furans, and polychlorinated biphenyls (PCBs, a group of toxic organic food contaminants)
These several hundred compounds are not new and have been present in the food chain for many years. New detection and analysis methods have made it possible to measure lower levels present in foods and people, and their impact on health. These compounds exist throughout the environment, almost every living creature, including humans. Eating food, primarily meat, dairy products, and fish, make up more than 90%

of dioxin intake for the general population. Dioxins are fat-soluble and accumulate in the fatty tissues of beef and dairy cattle, poultry, pork or seafood. Levels of dioxins tend to increase with age in these animals.

The World Health Organization has advised that long-term low-level exposure of humans to this group of compounds may lead to a weakened immune system, and the impaired development of the nervous system and the reproductive functions. Short-term high-level exposure could result in skin lesions and altered liver function.

5. Genetically Modified Foods

Genetically Modified (GM) refers to a special set of technologies that alter the genetic makeup of such living organisms as animals, plants, or bacteria. The technology combines genes from different organisms (recombinant DNA), and the resulting organism is said to be 'genetically modified', 'genetically engineered', or 'transgenic'.

The majority of the GM foods are produced in six countries: United States (63%), Argentina (21%), Canada (6%), Brazil (4%), China (4%), and South Africa (1%), and is spreading at increasing rates into the developing countries. Food sources include soya, cotton, canola, corn, meat and dairy products, and food additives (including the sweetener aspartame). The labelling of GM foods is mandatory in most developed countries, but interestingly, not in the United States.

There are many serious concerns about the environmental and health risks of this relatively new technology. There is already sufficient evidence to suggest that transgenic DNA in GM crops and products can spread by being taken up directly by viruses and bacteria, as well as plant and animals cells. Transgenic DNA has been is perfect for crossing from one organism or virus to another. This leads to the possibility of new recombined genetic compounds. The health risks include new viruses, allergens, and diseases, and if they reach the human cells, cause cancer. The risk of cancer is highlighted by the recent report that gene therapy - genetic modification of human cells – had claimed its first cancer victim.

6. Additives

In the early days, food additives were minimised to food items such as salt, sugar, and vinegar. The last few decades has seen an explosion of processed foods and the chemical adulteration of foods with additives. Controversy has been associated with the potential threats and possible benefits of food additives and will continue to do so. Most food additives are considered 'safe' while others have been proven carcinogenic or toxic to your body. As these chemical additives have only been extensively used in the last thirty years, there is always the risk that given further research and analysis, more additives will be added to the danger list. Conditions of hyperactivity in children, allergies, asthma, and migraines are often associated with adverse reactions to food additives.

Is saving time and added convenience a health hazard?
If you were to eat predominantly local fresh seasonal produce and invest your time into cooking and preparing it yourself, there would be no need for additives. Additives are added to food for mainly commercial reasons and fall under three main categories, with the aim to:

1. prolong shelf-life
2. replace nutrients, processing or poor farming, will have removed
3. improve the taste, texture, and appearance of 'unreal' packaged foods

The food industry will provide many 'health' related reasons as to why there is a need for additives in food, such as to:

- slow product spoilage caused by mould, bacteria, etc
- help control contamination
- prevent food from becoming rancid or developing an off-flavour
- prevent fruits like apples from turning brown when exposed to air
- fortify food with vitamins, minerals, or fibre
- enhance the taste of food
- maintain or improve appearance
- give foods the texture and consistency
- assist baked goods to rise during baking
- help control the acidity and alkalinity of foods
- maintain the taste and appeal of foods with reduced fat content

E Numbers and additives
There are over a thousand food additives. Food labels in most industrialised countries indicate when additives are used. Sometimes the labels will show the chemical names and other times just an E-number (which corresponds to an internationally recognised additive listing). The numbers range from E100 - Curcumin to E1520 - Propan-1,2-diol (propylene glycol) and continue to expand. The United Kingdom Food Standards Agency publishes a listing of E numbers split into major additive categories (colours, preservatives, etc). This can be found in the appendices section of this book, along with a listing of commonly found additives. Here are ten additives, which give you an idea of the dangers involved in consuming them.

Additive	No.	Use	Reasons to avoid
Aspartame	E951	Sweetener in snacks, sweets, alcohol, desserts, diet foods	Increase risks of headaches in the short term; and blindness and seizures in the long-term
Benzoic acid	E210	Preservative in many foods, including drinks, low sugar products, cereals, meat products	Inhibit the function of digestive enzymes. Adversely affect suffers of asthma, rhinitis, urticaria, or other allergies
Butylated Hydroxy-anisole	E320	Preservative, particularly in fat-containing foods, confectionery, meats	Possibly carcinogenic to humans, and interacts with nitrites, which go on to damage DNA cells.
Calcium sulphite	E226	Preservative in a vast array of foods-from burgers to biscuits, from frozen mushrooms to horseradish; Used to make old produce look fresh	Banned in many countries, sulphites; can cause bronchial problems, flushing, low blood pressure, tingling, and anaphylactic shock. Adversely affect suffers of bronchial asthma, cardiovascular or respiratory problems, and emphysema.
Monosodium glutamate (MSG)	E621	Flavour enhancer	Cause pressure on the head, seizures, chest pains, headache, nausea, burning sensations, and tightness of face.
Potassium benzoate	E212	Preservative in many foods, including drinks, low-sugar products, cereals, meat products	Can inhibit function of digestive enzymes; deplete amino acids. Adversely affect suffers of hay fever, hives, and asthma.

Parabens	F216	Preservative in cereals, snacks, pate, meat products, confectionery	Parabens have been identified as the cause of chronic dermatitis in numerous instances.
Saccharin	E954	Sweetener in diet, and no-sugar products	Saccharin is possibly carcinogenic to humans.
Sunset Yellow FCF, Orange Yellow S	E110	Food colouring	Some animal studies have indicated growth retardation. Adversely affect suffers of asthma, rhinitis, or urticaria.
Tartrazine	E102	Yellow food colouring	Cause allergic reactions and asthmatic attacks. Implicated in hyperactivity disorders in children; Adversely affect suffers of asthma, rhinitis, and urticaria.

7. Process-induced toxicants

Although the aim of cooking foods is to make them more appetising and microbiologically safe, it is now known that cooking and food processing at high temperatures such as frying, grilling, or baking generates various kinds of its own toxic substances, such as heterocyclic amines and acrylamide. Until recently, tobacco smoke was the major source of acrylamide, now it can be found in foods such as meat, potatoes, cereals, and coffee. In a study, the United States National Center for Environmental Health, Centers for Disease Control and Prevention, when assessing the human exposure to acrylamide, observed that the acrylamide found in foods had concentrations that exceeded the levels of other environment contaminants, such as pesticides.

The toxicity of acrylamide is under constant investigation. The major findings of these studies indicate that acrylamide is neurotoxic in animals and humans, and it has been shown to be a reproductive toxicant and carcinogen. The HEATOX project is a European Union project with thirty different partners, researching the health risks from heat-treated foods and food products, which have indicated that acrylamide and its by-products, produce an 'enhanced viability and malignancy to genetically compromised cells'.

8. Bacterial toxins

The battleground for bacterial toxins is in the home and workplace. There is a constant fight against, the known and unknown, bacterial toxins by ensuring high hygiene standards. Sanitation procedures and proper food treatment will help to keep you healthy. One such health-damaging toxin is produced by Clostridium botulinum (C. botulinum) and consumption of foods containing this neurotoxin will result in foodborne botulism. This foodborne intoxicant has been found in a considerable variety of foods, such as the canned foods: corn, peppers, green beans, soups, beets, asparagus, mushrooms, ripe olives, spinach, and tuna fish; chicken and chicken livers and liver pate; luncheon meats, ham, sausage; stuffed eggplant; and some seafood.

Only the smallest of amounts are necessary to cause intoxication and symptoms such as weakness and vertigo, double vision and progressive trouble in speaking and swallowing, difficulty in breathing, weakness of other muscles, abdominal problems, and constipation. Moreover, if not detected early enough the mortality rates are relatively high as the neurotoxin causes paralysis by blocking motor nerve terminals. The paralysis progresses downward, usually starting with the eyes, face, until the diaphragm and chest muscles are involved, then respiration is inhibited, and death from asphyxia results.

Mycotoxin is a fungal toxin; this has been around since the Sixties and is more commonly referred to as 'mould'. In some cases, the common mould produces a major mycotoxin called aflatoxin, which has been shown to cause chronic diseases such as, cancer, kidney toxicity, immune suppression, and death to those who are exposed to it.

There are some four hundred different mycotoxin compounds and the disease is referred to as mycotoxicosis, which can affect both animal and human food; opening a path from farm animals to, in a modified form, humans. Consuming food, which has become mouldy, increases your potential exposure to illness and disease.

9. Antibiotics

Most people have been prescribed antibiotics at some point in their lives. Since their discovery, there has been a growing use of antibiotics in the treatment of human illnesses and farming practices. On the farm, they are used on all types of animals from pigs to chickens and cows to fish. The three main reasons for their use are to treat ill animals; reduce illness and infection risks; and increase growth rates.

There has been evidence to show that the routine and overuse of these antibiotics can cause resistance to the life-saving antibiotics used in human medicine, to the point that some countries have selective bans in place preventing their use in farming. The banning of some antibiotics though is seen to be of little benefit, as the banned products, due to their profitability to the farmer, are just replaced by another similar antibiotic and their use on the farm continued.

There is no programme in place, which identifies antibiotic resistant bacteria in food, despite the fact that this was called for and identified as a serious issue. Resistant bacteria are present in food, farms (where it is extensively used) and in surrounding areas, so the food chain is attacked from all angles. The United Kingdom government has shown that there was conclusive evidence that the practice of antibiotic use in farming was helping to create 'superbugs' that threatened human health.

10. Parasitic infections

A parasite is any organism that lives at the expense of another (host) organism. Some parasites carry or cause disease. Parasites are a worldwide major health problem ranking amongst the greater threats to the well-being of people.

Parasitic infections are acquired by eating or drinking contaminated food or water, through direct contact with soil or water containing parasites or their larva, or by contact with biting insects. Parasitic infections have been a problem before, and it was thought to be under control. However, it has re-emerged as a health concern in developed countries, such as the United States, the Americas, and Europe, while continuing to be a major concern for many parts of the world. Food is a major vehicle for human parasites, and studies have shown many foodborne outbreaks associated with food, and here is just a sample of such items: ice cream, fruit, fish, imported vegetables, and chicken salad.

Millions are affected worldwide, and in the United States, the latest survey of foodborne illnesses by the Centers for Disease Control and Prevention estimates that there are 2.5 million cases annually due to food and beverage-borne parasites. This re-emergence and increase in parasitic infections has coincided with the increase in ease of international travel, the global distribution of food, and reduced individual immunity. The future will be further complicated by the emergence of new parasites, which have not so far been identified with pathogenesis in people.

Your food safety responsibility

By observing a strict policy of 'freshness' and 'safe food handling' at home and work will help you to avoid (only) four of the Top Ten 'Poisons on a plate'; these are: Foodborne bacterial and viral infections; Bacterial toxins; Antibiotics; and Parasitic infections.

The Three C's to health and safety:

Clean

- Wash hands and utensils thoroughly before and after use
- Ensure clean surfaces
- Clean fruit and vegetables before use
- Keep raw food (especially meat, poultry, and seafood) separate from cooked food
- Use separate utensils (chopping boards, knifes, containers, etc.) for foods such as meat, poultry, seafood, and fruit and vegetables

Cook

- Consume cooked foods immediately
- Reheat already cooked foods before eating
- Take special care with food containing meat, poultry, and seafood
- Avoid 'deli' style cold meats, uncooked meat, ready-to-eat foods, mussels, soft cheese and unpasteurised milk, cheeses, etc.
- Do not leave foods uncovered and exposed for long periods

Contain

- Refrigerate foods before preparation and cooking
- Use meat, poultry, and seafood on the day it is purchased
- Consume all foods within expiry dates
- Minimise use of refrigerator and freezer (using fresh foods and cooking foods on the purchase days)
- If foods need to be stored then they should be safely packed in containers to ensure freshness and avoid cross contamination
- Avoid leaving exposed or uncovered foods in the refrigerator

How to reduce the other six poisons-on-a-plate

There is a one-word answer to avoid the other six poisons from entering your food and damaging your health and well-being, and that word is 'local'. Seek and find locally grown and produced foods free from pesticides, additives, genetic modification, antibiotics, and toxicants. Organic farms and its produce are one example of such foods but not the only ones. There is a need to redress the alarming rates with which foods have gradually been depleted of essential minerals. In a 2006 study published in Food Magazine it was shown that since the 1930's mineral losses in foods were reported as: milk (iron reduced by 62%), cheddar cheese (magnesium reduced by 38%), turkey (calcium reduced by 71%), and chicken meat roast (iron reduced by 69%). Your average supermarket has begun to take organic foods more seriously, but will still actively source there organic stock from overseas suppliers, and thereby cancelling out any benefit gained from eating the organic food with an increase of environmental damage and pollution, which effectively increases other health risks.

Global trade and emerging infections was the subject of a study by Ann Marie Kimball and her fellow researchers at the University of Washington, Seattle, USA. It examined the link between the rapid expansion of global trade and the emergence and dissemination of new 'stealth' infections with long, silent incubation periods such as Human Immunodeficiency Virus (HIV) or variant Creutzfeld Jacob Disease (vCJD). It was shown that where global trade transports large volumes of diverse products to broad geographic areas of the world, that when emergent infections enter this system their transmission is amplified. This could open the door to truly novel emergent infections with long incubation periods, and silently disseminate the infection to far distant populations prior to detection.

Sourcing locally will reduce the risks of 'stealth' infections, as well as, the environmental damage and pollution caused by the expanding global transportation of food, such as that caused by the supermarket companies when importing their foods from other countries. Reduce the time from farm to fork, and taste the difference with nutrient packed foods of vast varieties, best flavours, and natural colours that have been around in your communities for many years. You will also be building and sustaining your community while proactively ensuring the big open spaces and agricultural landscape in the surrounding areas; providing local jobs for local people, continued local investment and reinvestment in small businesses, which will guarantee a diverse range of quality product choices.

'You get what you pay for' is a common saying and one especially true of the food you purchase. Industrial food and farming practices hide or obscure the hidden social, ecological, and human health costs of chemical and energy-intensive agriculture and animal factory farms. The pollution and public health damage resulting from massive toxic pesticide and fertiliser use, sweatshop conditions for workers, water pollution from agriculture runoff, and billions in taxpayer subsidies that mainly go to a handful of rich corporate farmers are not reflected in the price paid at the supermarket checkout. Given the hidden costs of industrial agriculture and long-distance food transportation, fair prices for local farmers (such as organic farmers) and farm workers are a bargain investment in your continued good health and well-being.

Furthermore, the overall cost of buying quality local food may be seen as more expensive than choosing the less expensive one in your supermarket. However, this is an artificially produced situation and the true costs of purchasing the quality and locally sourced foods will actually represent better value for money in the long-term. The buying power of food industry giants, will artificially deflate the costs of wholesale food prices, by paying the farmers (who are presented with little choice) tiny amounts for their produce. This in turn, allows them to be able to recuperate their other incurred costs, which come from the food packaging, processing, transportation, and advertising. Even then, they will still be able to under price their food products in comparison to smaller local suppliers. However, the fact is that you will require less quantity of the quality foods to fulfil your body's essential nutrient requirements than with the inferior supermarket product, and therefore, have to purchase and consume less of it, to receive the greater long-term benefits. So if it is value for money you are seeking (which is the factor, which drives most consumers), then buying locally sourced seasonal produce is the best value of all.

By having an idea of where your food comes from and how it is grown, will ensure not only quality food, but is a great way to develop your own food culture and relationships with the people providing it. Industrial food is bred for cosmetic perfection, long-distance travel, and longevity on the supermarket shelves. It is not just the growers and producers of food you need to be wary of, but also the meals eaten in restaurants, canteens, fast food outlets, and street level vendors. You should be extremely choosey about where you eat out, as the boom in food service establishments is not matched by the essential food health and safety. Unhygienic preparation of food provides many opportunities for contamination, growth, mutation, or survival of foodborne poisons. The advice is to prepare and enjoy your locally sourced food at home and in the workplace, or seek out establishments with a proven health and safety track record and stay loyal to them. Asking to inspect the food preparation area of a prospective establishment is the least you should do before having the confidence to eat there. Remembering that illness is an unpleasant experience at any time, but having to pay for the 'privilege' is just adding insult to injury.

What should you do? Get involved. Even if it is only by buying from local producers, as loyalty to quality local foods and establishments is the key to a vibrant community. You should value your food and the people who produce it, as your quality of life, and the reduction of the 'poisons on your plate' depends on it. You should also aim to be an active part of your community and seek out websites, organisations, local initiatives, and campaigns to help remove the existing and emerging dangers of the food poisons. As the next generation of food issues, are happening right now...

Fantasy foods - The next generation
At first, it was insecticides and pesticides; then the genetically modified foods; and now you are consuming and about to consume foods from the third generation. These biotechnologies are already surrounded by enormous hype, as the chemical giants unleash their mighty marketing machines on the consumer. The third generation food companies will look to use the negative experiences suffered from the first two-generation food controversies, and look to introduce a 'softer' consumer friendly approach in which 'health' comes first. Will it really be about consumer health though? On the other hand, will it be another attempt of food companies, with the help of the sciences, to distract people from eating healthy 'real' foods packed with multiple nutrients and encourage them to consume inferior foods with little or no value, other than the fact they contain one or other nutrient.

Coming soon to a supermarket near you; a host of new foods straight out of the science laboratory, with names such as functional foods, nutraceuticals, biotech foods, pharmafoods, and designer foods. Functional food incorporates many other descriptions of foods, which have essentially been specifically formulated to contain higher levels of nutrients, and non-nutrients that may incorporate some health benefits. All the major players, the food conglomerates, health food companies, biotechnology, and pharmaceutical giants are in place to profit from a rapidly expanding billion-dollar industry.

The food scientists have discovered the many health benefits derived from food such as carrots, apples, broccoli, soybeans, and their nutrients and non-nutrients such as phytochemicals (beta-carotene, isoflavones, and flavonoids), they contain. The phytochemicals are not necessary for life but they help to promote optimal health by lowering risk of chronic diseases, such as cancer and heart disease. They are found only in plant foods, with fruits and vegetables among the best sources of these compounds.

In the past, foods were commonly fortified with nutrients to help prevent specific nutritional deficiencies in an era when there was not the wealth of foods there are available today. Milk, for example, was fortified with vitamin D that was introduced in the 1930's to prevent rickets and continues to this day to be fortified and enriched. Technically, any fortified or enriched food is a functional food and there are many examples, orange juice fortified with calcium, salt fortified with iodine, and cereals, breads, and flours fortified with vitamins and minerals, and probiotic yoghurts.

Functional foods are sometimes called 'nutraceuticals' which comes from the two words 'nutrition' and 'pharmaceuticals' and is the process of taking these elements found naturally in fruits, vegetables, and some animal products and combining them within everyday foods such as:

- margarine spread, yogurt, and yogurt drinks with reducol
- cereals and breads with added isoflavones
- fruit juices with echinacea

According to an expert report by the Institute of Food Technologists, the functional and nutraceutical foods have spawned new science fields such as the disciplines nutrigenomics, proteomics and metabolomics, and the integration of genomics and nutrition, to help understand how a functional food affects health. The added 'expertise' however, does not stop the fact that some functional foods send out confusing and conflicting health messages such as calcium-fortified sweets, fibre-enriched white bread, and beer with added vitamin B, where science is used to add a beneficial substance to foods that are otherwise lacking in healthy properties.

Manufactured functional foods cannot duplicate all of the benefits of whole plant foods, some of which are not yet known. 'Real' foods that are consumed in their natural state (like fruits, vegetables, nuts, seeds, and grains) will naturally contain the nutrients essential for normal body functions and the non-essential nutrients which been shown to deliver many health benefits and disease fighting properties. Leafy green vegetables, for example, are naturally rich in calcium; and also provide vitamin K and vitamin C, numerous nutrients and phytochemicals that protect against chronic disease. A diet based on plant foods is likely to be more healthful than one based on functional foods.

Nanotechnology foods
Nanotechnology is the next stage up from functional foods and nutraceuticals and has promised a new 'nano' industrial revolution in nearly all economic sectors but especially the food and agriculture one.

Nanotechnology is the science of the extremely tiny. It involves the study and use of materials on an unimaginably small scale. A company in Japan, for example utilising nanotechnology, has succeeded in making ultra fine food particles small enough that once eaten will be able to pass through the walls of a person's intestines (this product was launched in December 2003). Japan is one of the top four players in the multi billion dollar nanotechnology industry, the others being the United States (the leader in the field), China, and the European Union. A recent study, from the Helmuth Kaiser Consultancy predicts that the nanotechnology food market will surge from $2.6 billion to $20.4 billion by 2010. Given these figures, it is not surprising that the global food giants Nestle, Kraft, Heinz, and Unilever are in place and devoting time and money into food nanotechnology to ensure their slices of the profits.

Nanotechnology is already being used today in the development of functional foods; nanoparticles are added to foods to increase effectiveness of enriched or fortified foods once inside the body. Companies around the world are working on new generation 'nano' food products, which respond to your body's requirements and deliver the appropriate levels of nutrients to your cells, or remain stored until they are required later. Foods can have vitamins and other non-essential nutrients added to them without changing their colour or taste, and the consumer having any knowledge that they are there. The way vitamins operate are also being altered; BASF AG, a global chemical company is internationally distributing a fat-soluble vitamin C (naturally a water-soluble one), which was developed and patented by AQUANOVA, with an agreement in place on a water-soluble vitamin E (naturally a fat-soluble one), with many other similar characteristic changing products on the way.

The nanotechnology foods are available now, include bread with tuna fish oil, where the fish oil is in the nanoparticles (so it carries no smell or taste), and will break-up only when they reach your stomach. In Canola Activa oil, where the makers of the oil claim it can reduce the cholesterol uptake of the body using the nanoparticles as, in effect, 'protectors'. A major food company is researching ways in which nanotechnology can be used to allow consumers to interact with their food by changing the colour and taste of it. In addition, develop foods which have sensors and capsules within them, and these 'smart' foods will lay dormant in your body until activated. They say the foods will offer the potential benefits of increased energy, improved brain functions, boosted immune system, and a way to fight aging. The same researchers are also studying the possibility of 'intelligent weight management' foods where nanoparticles are deployed to fight the storing of body fat and increase satiety at the same time.

Is your health and safety compromised?
The complex and intricate nature of the 'nano' foods will represent an overwhelming challenge for the government health and safety agencies to ensure the appropriate regulatory measures are in place to protect consumers. As previously mentioned there are already products out there, which have been manufactured by, or contain components of the nanotechnology industry being bought and sold in the world economy. These 'nano' food products will continue to be manufactured and licensed, as they will conveniently fall into the food 'supplement' category which has much less government regulation than the drug sector for example. The food industry (with the drug industry taking a

close look at the new developments) will continue to grow and compromise your health and safety until the, inadvertent experiment participants, the consumers, has reported in large enough numbers that there are adverse effects of the 'nano' foods. There are no tests or standards in place to identify the new toxicological risks posed by the new 'nano' foods with the government agencies (such as the United States Food and Drug Administration) assuming that existing regulations will be adequate to cover these new nanotechnology products.

Do yourself and your family a just service and try not to become part of the food scientist's experiments. Do not be sucked in by the supposedly fantastic nutritional benefits of these products that will be trumpeted loudly and proudly by the food industry moneymaking machines. Keep your food real.

Chapter 10

Food for thought

How can you use this vast pool of nourishment knowledge? The following Food Intake Guidelines are devised to offer you the way to maximise your health benefits while reducing your risks of developing heart and cardiovascular disease, hypertension, some cancers, obesity, type 2 diabetes, osteoporosis, premature aging, and debilitating illnesses.

> Most illnesses arise solely from long-continued errors of diet and regimen.
>
> *Ibn Sina (Avicenna); 980-1037AD*

Ibn Sina, often referred to, by his Latin name Avicenna, was a great Iranian physician and scholar, known as the Prince of Physicians in the Persian Empire. He was born 980AD in a place called Buhara, and from an early age started to study human health, at first from his father and then from the masters of that time. At the age of seventeen, Ibn Sina cured the Prince of Buhara from a life-threatening illness, and gratitude, took the shape of a great library in the Buhara palace. In 1012AD, he began writing his great medical text Al-Qanun fi'l at-Tibb (The Canon of Medicine) when completed; it was translated from Arabic into Latin, and it formed the foundation of medicine in Europe.

The Prophet Muhammad is known to have summed up the teaching of Ibn Sina regarding good health when he said 'The stomach is the home of disease, diet is the main medicine'. Words of wisdom about the relationship between illness and diet have been around for over a thousand years and geography could not stem the flow of knowledge as at around the same time the Chinese were teaching that 'Whatsoever was the father of disease, an ill diet was the mother'.

These teachings, despite being over a thousand years old, are not outdated and stand tall, like beacons of light to those who wish to pursue a healthy lifestyle today.

Food intake guidelines

> Your body is the baggage you must carry through life.
> The more excess you carry, the shorter the trip.
> *Arnold H. Glasgow*

The guidelines draw on knowledge from the past and present, and in concert with the latest research and clinical studies, point you in the direction of a healthier lifestyle. You need to think of a healthy lifestyle and your food intake as a journey and not a burden or chore; an adventure which is full of discovery and creation, where each step will bring you closer to the kind of healthy lifestyle you are looking for. Of course, there will be the occasions when you veer off course, but as long as you acknowledge the benefits of the Food Intake Guidelines, and realise it is an organic process, in which small daily steps will infuse their way into your lifestyle, you will continue to follow them and continue to head in the right general direction. In taking these small positive steps, you will be moving closer towards good health, and reaping the rewards in the short and long-term.

The Food Intake Guidelines are summed up by the acronym FITTTT or just **FIT**[4].

- Frequency
- Ingredients
- Timing - Taste - Treat - Thankful

Frequency

Irregular eating habits can have an impact on your future health. In recent studies by the Institute of Clinical Research at the University of Nottingham, researchers investigated the impact of regular meal frequencies on various factors, which are known to increase the risks of cardiovascular disease, and increased body weight. The results showed that irregular eating patterns produced inappropriate insulin sensitivity and a detrimental effect on cholesterol ratios, and decreased thermic effects, which can all be factors for an increased risk of obesity, type 2 diabetes, and cardiovascular diseases.

Supplementing your main three meals a day with additional 'bite-size' type meals, as long as your activity levels require the extra energy, have been associated with participants who had better body compositions (lower body fat levels and increased lean body mass). However, as shown in the study published in the International Journal of Obesity, it is important that you match the frequency of your meals to your activity rates, as eating more than three meals per day, with the extra calories consumed, will only lead to an increase in weight, and the continued over consumption will increase the risks of obesity.

- Avoid missing meals
- Aim for three regular meals
- Supplement with one to three 'bite-size meals' per day; dependant on your energy needs.
- Always carry a 'bite-size meal' wherever you go. E.g., Fruit, nuts, and seeds; easily carried and full of all major nutrients, especially when:
  - busy and always-on-the-go
  - food options are limited and/or of poor quality

Ingredients

> Research shows that diseases of almost every variety can be produced by an under-supply of various combinations of nutrients... [And] can be corrected when all nutrients are supplied...
>
> *Adelle Davis*
> *Author of Let's Get Well - 1965*

Adelle Davis was an American pioneer in the field of nutrition, and an outspoken advocate of the superior value of whole unprocessed foods, highlighting the dangers of food additives, and the dominant role that all nutrients play in maintaining health, preventing disease, and restoring health after the onset of disease. Her message is as true in her days as it is now, and 'Ingredients' are the focus of the next Food Intake Guideline.

Quality of the food is the number one factor. Seek and find locally grown and produced foods free from pesticides, additives, genetic modification, antibiotics, and toxicants. Organic farms and its produce are one example of such foods but not the only ones, as there are now increasing numbers of farmers, producers and retailers, which cater for 'real' food, for people who wish to eat quality nourishing, repairing, and rejuvenating food.

The MaxLife70 foods, which satisfy these criteria, should form the basis for the foods you purchase and consume. These foods have proven health benefiting macro and micronutrients. The first step is to maximise your intake of the MaxLife7 Super foods and incorporate them often into your daily food intake (when seasonally available), to experience the amazing natural life preserving and regenerating properties stored in them. Your aim is to consume the majority of your food from the Fruits; Vegetables (and Herbs); Beans & Legumes; Whole grains; and the Nuts, seeds, & oils groupings and reap the optimum health harvest. Ideally, an appropriate quantity from each of these groups at every meal would be perfect. For the average person food quantities should be roughly gauged on a sliding quantity scale:

Fruits; Vegetables (and Herbs) - 5 to 6 daily servings
Beans; Legumes; Whole grains - 4 to 5 daily servings
Nuts; Seeds; Oils   - 3 to 4 daily tablespoon serving
The Occasionals   - 1 to 2 daily moderate servings

Also, reduce your weekly food intake from The Occasionals grouping (milk, cheese, meat, poultry, fish, eggs, and desserts). Most of these foods carry high levels of saturated fats, cholesterol, and other factors, which interfere with your journey to good health. You should limit your intake to one item from the list per day. And there is no need to worry about your protein levels, as you only need moderate daily levels of protein to receive the maximum benefits they offer; and all the essential amino acids your body requires per day will be adequately supplied by the beans, legumes, whole grains, nuts, seeds, and vegetables you will be eating.

> One-fourth of what you eat keeps you alive
> The other three-fourths keep your doctor alive
> *Egyptian writing found on a tomb wall*

Portion size is a potent determinant of how much a person eats, regardless of the size of the meal you eat; there is not that much difference to be felt in how full you feel or how hungry you will be later on. Not only will larger portion sizes increase your total calorie intake and put you on the road to increased body weight, but also you will also not feel any fuller or less hungry in the process.

In recent studies at the Nutrition Department, of Pennsylvania State University, it was shown that reduced portion sizes (and lower energy dense foods such as fruits, vegetables, whole grains, etc.) maintained levels of satiety and reduced the overall intake of the participants without any signs of increased hunger. In one of the clinical trials, advising individuals to eat portions of lower energy dense foods was a more successful weight loss strategy than fat reductions in food or restricting portion sizes. The research concluded that eating satisfying portions of lower energy dense foods could help to enhance satiety and control hunger while restricting energy intake for weight management.

- Seek and find local and seasonal high quality foods
  - Leading to more nutrients and less quantity of the quality foods per meal (this equals an increased economy and a better investment in your health)
- Ensure weekly consumption of the MaxLife7 Super foods
- Choose foods on the MaxLife70 shopping list

- o The majority of your foods should come from: Fruits; Vegetables (and Herbs); Beans; Legumes; Whole grains; supplemented by Nuts; Seeds; Oils
- Prioritise lower energy dense foods (fruits, vegetables, beans, legumes, whole grains) to:
  - o increase your feeling of fullness
  - o decrease hunger
  - o maximise nutrient uptake
  - o improve appetite and weight management control
- Replace saturated fats and trans fatty acids with the healthier fats:
  - o Polyunsaturated fats
  - o Monounsaturated fats
- Cut back on processed, packaged, junk, and fast foods; and also The Occasionals food group, to reduce the:
  - o saturated fats & trans fatty acids (hydrogenated & partially hydrogenated fats)
  - o excess salt consumption
  - o cholesterol intake
  - o simple sugar and artificial sweetener quantities
  - o exposure to some 'poisons on a plate'
- Minimise cooking, and where possible:
  - o eat fruits and vegetables in their natural states
  - o steam, stir-fry, sauté, roast your food

Timing

> Eat breakfast like a king, lunch like a prince, and dinner like a pauper.
>
> *Adelle Davis*

'Breakfast is the most important meal of the day' and boasts plentiful research that lends credibility to this often-repeated advice. Is the advice being followed? By fewer and fewer people is the answer. In the report, 'The Future of Mealtimes' compiled by the market analyst Datamonitor, they reveal that breakfast is 'the most missed meal in Europe'. Europeans skip 18% of their breakfasts, while the British consumers will miss 30% of their morning meals. And the future is no brighter as the report goes on to predict that by 2009, British consumers will consume less main meals at home with breakfast being the most frequently missed meal. The American consumers fair no better; in a recent article in the LA Times, it was reported that Americans skip 30% of their breakfasts.

The Third National Health and Nutrition Examination Survey (NHANES III), 1988-94, was conducted on a nationwide probability sample of 33,994 participants. It found that breakfast skippers are more likely to gain weight, because they are more inclined to overcompensate for the loss of key nutrients at breakfast by eating more fat-rich, high-energy foods, later in the day. In another more recent study, the American Journal of Clinical Nutrition concluded that not having breakfast resulted in a damaging effect on insulin sensitivity and cholesterol levels in the experiment participants. While in the Journal of Nutrition, having a good breakfast was particularly satiating, and could reduce the total amount of food eaten for the rest of the day.

'Eating late at night or just before you sleep will make you fat' is another piece of 'advice' often given but it turns out to be nothing more than a myth; and in dispelling it you discover one of the keys to understanding and combating weight gain. The timing of late night meals are irrelevant when it comes to putting on weight or not. It is often said, that food eaten just before you go to sleep will not be properly digested and will be stored as fat. This is just not the case, and the National Institutes of Health, which is the United States Federal Government's lead agency responsible for biomedical research on nutrition and obesity, will support this statement. It is important to realise that it is how much food that you eat (total energy intake) counter balanced by your body needs and how much physical activity (total energy expenditure) you do during the whole day that determines whether you gain, lose, or maintain your weight. So eating before you sleep compared with any other time of day, does not increase the chance of it being stored as fat.

This said you have to be aware of a couple of points highlighted in the research by John M. de Castro at the University of Texas and his study concerning the 'The Time of Day of Food Intake Influences Overall Intake in Humans'. Your level of satiety or the feeling of fullness has been shown to decrease as the day progresses, and you are drawn into eating higher calorie foods and reducing the gap between meals. There are many physiological mechanisms and psychological characteristics, which affect food intake. The exact reason, as to why a person's satiety reduces over the day has so far eluded researchers but they predict that it is part of the human survival instinct and body rhythms. Historically your instincts may have propelled you into eating more ahead of sleep (an enforced fasting period), as a safeguard against not knowing where the next meal may come from the next day. The study also associated very late meal times with an increase of total calories over the course of the day, which suggests people are more likely to binge on foods that are high in sugar, salt, and fat.

If you maintain regular mealtimes with gaps approximately three to four hours between them and eat high quality foods, it will improve your satiety throughout the day and reduce the total amount of calories consumed. This will increase your appetite control and weight management, while also avoiding the increased risks of being overweight or obese, and improve your blood sugar, insulin balance, and sensitivity.

The speed at which you eat also affects your health and in a recent study, Japanese researchers were curious as to whether how fast a person eats has any effect on how much they weigh, as its population has been gaining weight steadily over the past few decades. More than 5,000 employees with age ranges from 35 to 69 were involved in study. The results showed that the faster you ate the more likely it was you would be overweight or obese. This was represented by a positive correlation between the speeds of eating and body weight.

Taste

A mouthful spent of treasure, is a pleasure

Health-Warrior

Sensory factors are important determinants of appetite and food choice from birth to old age, and there is no doubt that your physiological make-up draws you to certain tastes, such as sweet, salt, and fat; and once upon a time human survival may have depended on it. Humans are instinctually drawn to sweet flavours, and the consuming of fats has been shown to release brain receptors similar to the ones in reaction to the drug morphine. However, in the main humans do not have the same survival needs as they did then; it is not a case of feast or famine, as most people now, have an abundance of food. There is much evidence to show that sugar has the similar addictive properties and brain wave patterns as drug use does. While other studies show that consuming many varieties of opposing flavours in meals leads to excess stimulation and the overeating of food. If you are to avoid altering your central nervous system functions with excessive quantities of addictive substances, such as those experienced with sugar and fat, then you need to take a closer look at the physiology involved in eating food.

When you eat food, to enjoy it and its differing flavours you need to try to experience it through as many of your senses as you can. The taste, smell, and feel of foods are an important part of the process of food selection and consumption; and the further processes of ingestion, energy production, and maintaining your body perfectly balanced with the nutrients it needs.

Your tongue can distinguish between thousands of differing flavours and your numerous taste buds, which are renewed every ten days or so, will only be activated when food is dissolved in your mouth by the joint effects of your teeth and saliva. You have the ability to recognise four different taste groupings: sweet, sour, salty, and bitter. Sugar by far has the highest taste threshold; for instance, you can consume sugary products in large quantities without provoking unpleasant reactions, whereas, bitter tastes have very low thresholds, which can turn you off, soon after eating relatively tiny amounts. Salty and sour thresholds sit between sweet and bitter.

The smell of foods is important in detecting flavours but also in regulating appetite and food intake (for example, the loss of appetite you experience when you had a 'blocked' nose during a cold). Smell can also evoke strong attraction or avoidance behaviours; think of the fantastic aroma of bread wafting from the bakery as an example of 'attraction' and the smell of rotting foods (such as an egg) a good case for 'avoidance'. The smell of attractive food will get the digestive juices flowing, and when you eat, the aromas from the food travel up into your nasal passages, especially after breaking up the food during chewing.

Lastly, the sense of touch, the hardness, texture, and consistency as you chew and move your food around. The feel of the food can be an important guide to flavour and quality of it. The temperature of the food is another factor in determining flavour. A food, which is overly hot or cold, will just mask its flavour and in general, people use the heating and cooling appliances of food far too freely, and with little regard for its true flavours.

To experience an expanded spectrum of food flavours you should:

- chew your foods thoroughly to release all available flavours
- use your senses such as taste, smell, and touch to heighten the eating experience
- utilise the full range of flavours from your food; sweet, salty, sour, and bitter (but not all at once)

The messages from food via the senses of a person are sent through a network of trillions of neurons and connectors to the limbic system. This area has an important role in your emotional state, memory formation, and conscious thought, so when taste messages arrive here, you experience pleasant, aversive, or other emotions, such as child memories of favourite foods.

Each brain cell relies on these messages to maintain a balanced (homeostasis) state to function properly. Eating 'real' foods will supply your cells with the nutrients and enzymes they require to maintain this balance. The problems start to occur when this balance is upset and the body's neurochemistry is altered.

Your diet can affect this brain balance and create urges, cravings, and addictions in your food behaviour. In has been shown that mood altering foods release the same neurotransmitter into the brain as do nicotine, caffeine, and illegal drugs such as cocaine and heroin. This neurotransmitter is called dopamine, and its studies are increasingly linking it with the behaviours associated with food addiction. Dopamine does however have an important role to play in the body; it is the pleasurable feeling you receive as reward (and reinforcement) of a behaviour. When you feel pleasure from eating, it is a sensation caused by dopamine. In the early days of the human, these chemical messages sent to the brain ensured (among other things) humans were rewarded for finding wholesome nutritious foods, such as the sugar (and small amounts of salt) found in fruits and vegetables, and the oils in nuts and seeds. When food was scarce and it was a matter of human survival then the good sensations provided by dopamine was a positive evolutionary adaptation. However, this originally positive adaptation has found a more sinister side, and opened doors to modern illnesses and diseases.

> …it may seem paradoxical, but it is certainly true, that in the long run the moderate man will derive more enjoyment even from eating and drinking, than the glutton or the drunkard will ever obtain.
>
> *Sir John Lubbock*

The consumption of foods, which have excessive amounts of sugar, salt, or fats, affects a body's balance (with similar imbalances as seen with the intake of caffeine) and they also release dopamine causing a pleasurable sensation or a drug-like food fix. Once the 'pleasure pathway' to the brain has been established, it can form powerful physical and emotional triggers, which compel you to repeat your behaviour. So powerful are the triggers that they can create desires and urges which override your basic energy needs. However, your body will seek to regain its natural balance, and over time, will alter the neurochemistry to adapt to high repetition of the artificial food 'highs'. It has been shown that the body will reduce the number of dopamine receptors which are there to receive the pleasurable sensation messages, and what this in effect does, is to reduce the 'high' you feel from that food.

Research conducted at the U.S. Department of Energy's Brookhaven National Laboratory in New York shows that there is a distinct lack of dopamine brain receptors in chronic binge and overeaters. Dr. Gene-Jack Wang led the studies investigating the brain chemistry of chronic overeaters and showed that the brains of obese people and drug addicts had similar characteristics; they had decreased dopamine receptors, reduced sensitivity to reward stimuli associated with consumption, and increased vulnerability to overcompensate (overuse or overeating).

The average chocolate bar is loaded with salt, sugar, caffeine, and fat. When you consume a bar of chocolate, you will experience the 'high' pleasure of a food-fix caused by dopamine. Your body will associate the bar of chocolate with the 'high' you felt when eating it, and lay down the 'pleasure pathway' that forms a food trigger. This trigger will create an urge for you to consume other bars of chocolate and receive the same 'high' as before. The chocolate bar overloads your senses (far above the levels of what your body's neurochemistry is made for) and if repeated often will lead to reduction in dopamine receptors, as your body fights to regain its chemical balance. This means that you will need to consume more of the chocolate bar in order to receive the same 'high' sensations as before. The more you consume the more the risk that these brain receptors are turned off and you are liable to descend the vicious spiral to addiction.

Repeated bingeing on large amounts of high sugar, salt, or fat filled foods creates cravings for each of those foods. They all promise satisfaction, but the artificial pleasure, which is devoid of essential nutrients will never satisfy you, and this 'high' is ultimately paid for with your health. You will never feel the same 'high' as you did the first time and you will be left undernourished and be overloaded with excess calories. The body cravings override (as any addiction will do) the natural needs of the body as it craves for the substances necessary for the 'high'. Like a body demanding drugs for its 'balance', the body will crave sugar, salt and fat. After an addiction has been created, any type of restriction will cause withdrawal symptoms, and total removal of the sugar, processed fat, or salt from your diet, and you will go through the discomfort of facing withdrawal symptoms similar to those suffered from drug addictions.

It has taken decades of hard work for the food industry scientists to figure out the right combination of ingredients to improve the 'hook' on consumers. In his book, The Flavor Point Diet, Dr. David L. Katz, director of the Yale-Griffin Prevention Research Center, details how the scientists have now excelled at hitting the 'craving-spot' and making a person want more and more of the food. Providing foods, which are there to overload your senses and lay the pathway to cravings and addiction, leading to chronic illnesses and eventually diseases.

Once upon a time, it may have been down to just a choice or preference in what you ate, but as you have seen, the 'choice' is slowly being levered out of your control. There are already many people who suffer from food eating disorders and drug addictions, therefore, it seems only a question of time until there are sugar, salt, and fat 'rehab' centres whose mission it is to treat a person's addiction and integrate suffers back into a healthier lifestyle. The chances of stopping the food industry and their health damaging foods and practices are remote. Therefore, you need to proceed with caution through the minefield of 'pleasure' foods and their effect on your health and well-being.

Treat
A treat can be viewed as a special food that tastes good, and one that you do not eat very often. You need to choose your treats with care as they can either lead you to a healthy nutritious lifestyle or fighting the up and downs of bingeing and over indulgence.

> Go to your banquet then, but use delight,
> So as to rise still with an appetite
>
> *Herrick*

What are your treats: bacon and eggs, sausage sandwich, steak and chips, fast food hamburger, milkshake, and fries or is it a kebab, curry and rice, beef chow mein, fried chicken or pizza? For some it may be a bar of chocolate, potato chips, biscuits, cookies, cheesecake, cake and custard, ice cream, pie and fresh cream, doughnuts, or cheese filled croissants? On the other hand, maybe it is a bowl of salty and savoury snacks while watching the TV: tortilla and corn and dips, pretzels, crackers and cheese, roasted peanuts, or assorted salty nuts. Whatever your treat is, it will elicit a food high and have certain triggers, which set the process into action.

It is unlikely there will ever be stampedes in the direction of the fruit bowl, or people feeling guilty about the apple binge before sleep, or the need for late night grocers to cater for the partygoers craving for half a kilo of strawberries. The idea is to make the treat just that, and one that is eaten occasionally; only then can you seek to enjoy the food pleasures without the negatives side-effects encountered by the artificial food 'highs'.

Your aim is to replace the majority of the nutrient-less and energy dense foods with alternatives (some of which are not necessarily lower in fat but do contain 'healthier' fats) which can offer the similar pleasures but without the side effects. Fruits, natural nuts, and seeds are such examples and offer a great combination of natural sugar, salt, and healthy fats. There are many more examples of 'real' foods which can easily replace the 'unhealthy' treats you have in your current regime such as dried fruit, water-based smoothies, frozen fruit desserts, low fat yoghurts, popcorn, home baked cakes or cookies, olive products, carob products, humus, peanut, sesame, and hazelnut pastes.

- Enjoy your treats!
- Eat your fair share (25%) of healthier fats
- Use 'real' food substitutes as your desired treats

- o This will satisfy your sugar, salt, or fat desire and help you to reduce binging on addictive junk foods
- Avoid and limit the portion size and frequency of high sugar, salt, and saturated fat foods

Thankful

Since the beginning of time, foods have been incorporated into the religious practices of people around the world. Some religious sects abstain, or are forbidden, from consuming certain foods and drinks; others restrict foods and drinks during their holy days; while still others associate dietary and food preparation practices with rituals of the faith. A common theme, which runs through all faiths or religions, having been passed down and preserved in scriptures and writings, is the gratitude or thanksgiving for food. You need to establish, and in some cases re-establish this gratitude for food.

Eating is an enjoyable experience and one that should not be shrouded in guilt, shame, or fear of food. Eating healthily is as natural as the growing and harvesting of the foods themselves, and the appreciation of food goes beyond just how it tastes. The process of eating takes a person from nature and the fulfilling of hunger, to nurture and the cultivation of a person's emotional, physical, and spiritual well-being.

> Nature can take care of our needs, but not necessarily our greeds.
>
> *Gandhi*

Most people in developed and developing countries live in cultures with an abundant supply of food; in fact, they are surrounded by it. How or where these foods come from is of little concern to most. This abundance is regularly over eaten, over-purchased, and stockpiled in excess of a person's needs, it is, therefore, difficult for people to really appreciate what it means or to show the desire to be thankful for their food.

The surplus of foods for some people is in stark contrast to the, in excess of, one billion people who live on the equivalent of $1 a day, and a similarly high number live in conditions of starvation or malnutrition around the world, according to the Food and Agriculture Organisation of the United Nations and the World Bank. This leads to the deaths of 30,000 people a day attributable to hunger, and represents an increase on the previous year. It is not just the concern of underdeveloped and developing nations; the United States government produced in a report entitled 'Household Food Security', and highlighted that over 38 million people (and rising) are living with the risk of hunger in 2004, and also highlighted an upward trend from the figures recorded in the previous year. To show an appreciation to food is to consume it in moderation and waste none. Wise words of Aristotle over two thousand years ago signposted the path to follow when he taught that excellence lay in the balance between two extremes. For your body to function at its optimum level you need to maintain this path of excellence, a path of moderation (see Part six - A silent revolution).

Be thankful and ensure care is taken to:

- prioritise your need and make the time for your food and nourishment, a special one
  - try to prepare your own foods
- avoid multi-tasking while eating
  - free of distractions (such as a TV or computer)
- take special care of where you choose to eat
  - eating should be a family affair
  - there should be set place of where you eat, and you should employ similar routines at each sitting
  - place all the food courses for that meal in front of you
- avoid negative eating
  - emotional eating; address the underlying problem
  - excessive concern, judgements, and anxiety about food
- find the path of excellence; a path of moderation
  - daily food purchases will help you consume and use less
  - rise from a meal before any feelings of fullness appear (you will rarely shown guilt or frustration at rising from the meal having eaten too little)
- begin and conclude any meal with silent reflection to appreciate the journey of your nourishment from the farm to your fork, and the importance of your meal on your continued good health and well-being

Chapter 11

Food fights

Everyday you are battling against well-oiled and well-funded industries and organisations for your health and well-being. Food trends and consumer behaviour continues to move towards unhealthy foods despite the overwhelming knowledge of the damage they can do to health. People are making themselves ill in the short-term and at increased risk of diseases in the long-term. Why would a person consciously choose to eat foods, which will eventually reduce quality of living and ultimately, shorten life?

In this chapter, you will explore why and how this is the case, and what forces are against you in your battle to regain your good health and well-being.

> There is a force in this country that's out to poison your food, to make it addictive, to manipulate your very body chemistry. This conspiracy wants to keep you overfed but undernourished. Who's behind this conspiracy? The food giants.
>
> *Paul Stitt*
> *author of Beating the Food Giants*

How do food companies tailor their products to make them more addictive for consumers when eaten? Flavour is one of the keys to the attractiveness of junk food. The food companies engineer the perfect blend of salt, sugar, and fat (saturated and trans fats), which when combined with taste and smell makes the food highly desirable, and illicit feel-good sensations. The 10,000 taste buds on your tongue and in your mouth can pick up the four basic tastes: salt, sour, sweet, and bitter. However, it is the human nose, which can distinguish about 20,000 odours in the tiniest amounts, and contributes more to your sense of flavour. Smell is a powerful sensation that helps to shape your psychology, is strongly linked to your memory; and it is this powerful combination, which makes people often return to "comfort food" without quite knowing why.

Addictive food
The food industry has been quietly working away in their expensive laboratories to make use of this kind of knowledge. All junk and fast foods are industrially processed; the processes legally add chemical colourings and flavourings to make the food more appeasing to your flavour sensors, and adjust the texture of the foods by adding ranges of saturated and trans fats, gums, starches, emulsifiers, and stabilisers to appeal to your sense of touch.

> Science behind the Brands: Many people think of P&G [Proctor & Gamble] as simply a marketing company and are surprised by the enormous depth and breadth of our science capability.
>
> *Proctor & Gamble*
> *owners of Pringles snacks*

The scientists have been very successful at this fine and intricate art, and the result of their chemistry is that for some people these foods have become addictive. These nutrient-less "addictive" foods carry high calories from the excessive amounts of refined sugar, salt, processed fats (saturated and trans fats), and chemicals; these foods have been shown to cause hormonal imbalances in your body which encourage overeating and increase your risks of illness and disease.

In a study published in the journal, Nature Clinical Practice Endocrinology and Metabolism, Professor Robert Lustig, from the University of California, showed that changes in manufacturing processes were making food 'toxic' and 'addictive'. He points at the fact that the way in which food is now processed has changed significantly in the last thirty years, and has created an environment in which foods are essentially addictive due to their high sugar content and the lack of healthy ingredients such as fibre. Adding that, the high sugar content of foods causes chemical adaptations in the brain, which encourage overeating, discourage activity, while rewarding the consumer by inducing the food 'high'. Professor Lustig points out that higher sugar content can now be found in a wide variety of foods, many more than in previous decades, increasing the risks of more addictive foods.

The Chicago Tribune went one-step further when it published a three-part exposé about the American cookies Oreo's, and investigated the role it played in the discovery of sugar's addictive qualities and in child obesity. It highlighted the fact that food companies like Kraft, which makes Oreos, have made massive efforts to figure out how and why consumers are attracted to their products, producing evidence of collusion with a tobacco company and consultants, to help understand the brain science behind why consumers are so stimulated when they eat sugar packed products. During this time, the Oreo cookie had a meteoric rise in popularity, and easily became the number one selling American cookie in the world.

Those times were good for Kraft Foods but a dark cloud was on the horizon, and the ride, more recently, has been a little bumpier. Pressure from a lawsuit requiring the banning of trans fats from the Oreo cookie range, the cessation of advertising to children, a new public health awareness of the dangers of trans fats, and a backlash from the obesity publicity pushed the Oreo (and overall cookie) sales downward. Kraft has been forced into direct adverts to children, manufacturing 'healthier' cookies, and their biggest expense, the reformulating of their entire product range to reduce trans fats from their ingredients, to meet the trans-fat labelling regulations put in place by the United States Food and Drug Administration on the 1st January 2006. Before this time, in just one biscuit, you were able to put away more than the recommended level of trans fats.

The new trans-fat-free Oreo cookies (as well as the numerous other Kraft products) hit the isles in January 2006. Independent tasters found (to the credit of the excellent scientists) very little difference between to the old and new versions of the cookie. They did however mention that there was a hint more salt in the taste but they had the same sweetness and mouth-feel to them. The new trans-fat-free Chocolate sandwich Oreo cookies, a renowned best seller, is sold in a pack of 24; in just three cookies they contain 160 calories, 7 total fat grams (2g saturated fat, 1g polyunsaturated fat, 3g monounsaturated fat, 1g unidentified fat?), 14 grams of sugar, and 160 mg of sodium. The Oreo however remains a high fat (nearly 38% of calorie total), high sugar (35%), and high salt (over 10% of your Food and Nutrition recommended Daily Adequate Intake). It is no surprise then, that the Oreo cookies are still the top sellers making over $250 million per year and represents a market leading company, which corners over 36% of the $5.6 billion cookie market.

Procter & Gamble launched Pringles in the United Kingdom in July 1991, and like the Oreo enjoyed mass appeal propelling it into the bestselling snack foods lists. It flourished behind a major worldwide advertising campaign, which claimed 'Once you pop you can't stop'.

Pringles ingredients: Dehydrated potatoes, vegetable oil, wheat starch rice flour, corn flour, maltodextrin, emulsifier E471, salt, and dextrose

Why is it 'Once you pop you can't stop'? All becomes clearer when you check the 'irresistible' formulation of the Pringles ingredients (above) and analyse the 'nutritional' content; in a 25g serving 61% of the total calories come from fat (over a third coming from saturated fat), 34% from simple carbohydrates [read sugar], and of course, salt and a touch of (more) sugar. Like the Oreo sales, Pringles were hit as people address concerns about healthy eating. A rethink at Proctor & Gamble introduced new products such as Pringles Reduced Fat (Light), Fat-Free and smaller packages. It also changed the once globally trumpeted advertising campaign 'Once you pop you can't stop' to 'Once you pop the fun don't stop'. The words may have changed (and will continue to change), but the nature of the product has not, and marketing ploys of introducing smaller packages or 'healthier' versions of junk food, is still junk. It does not address its effects on your body and health.

Researchers believe that the overeating effect could be triggered by opioids, chemicals that produce a desire to eat more while reducing the 'sated' feeling that normally kills appetite. Dr Martin Yeomans, of the University of Sussex, a leading authority on opioids, has shown that they can have a dramatic effect on food intake. According to a 20-year review of scientist's research and experiments, conducted at the University of Sussex, it was shown that when the release of opioids was blocked using drugs, food intake among human volunteers fell by 21%. The effect was even larger among obese participants, whose intake fell by 33%. Further research suggests that the opioids effect is strongest with products that involve certain combinations of foods. These foods are typically high in fat and sugar; such as the family favourites, milk and cookies, chocolate or biscuits; cheese and salty snacks; or burgers and sugar filled buns with ketchup or mayonnaise.

The knowledge of these reactions elicited in people to certain foods has been around for decades, and the food companies have had access to and received briefings from the scientists involved in these studies (employing some of them directly as consultants). Originally, the food companies may not have deliberately set out to produce addictive food but only to create foods that were more palatable to consumers in an attempt to ensure a profitable product. However, in the process they have created foods, which interfere with the body's ability to control intake and could be shown as one of the causes of the global obesity epidemic. This kind of revelation would require those people who think of the overweight and obesity issue as one where people lack discipline and willpower, or accuse the suffers of being greedy and gluttonous, to show more understanding.

As the research continues to mount against the food companies, they continue to rack up the sales and reap mega profits from junk and fast food products. According to PDR Family Guide to Nutrition and Health, the United States fast foods and snacks such as candy, sweets, chips, cookies, ice cream, biscuits, and cakes business is booming, and in 2004, companies registered over $27 billion sales. Nearly half of the Americans who eat out, a third of them will chose fast food.

For the United Kingdom, the figures are just as shocking with sales of £9 billion in 2003, with estimates showing years of continued growth ahead. Chocolate is the largest contributor to sales, followed by crisps and snacks (with relatively greater increases in savoury snacks). In the United Kingdom, convenience (packaged and processed) foods represented nearly £18 billion, nearly a third of total food expenditure and is in contrast to the sales of fruit and vegetables which only attracted £10.72 billion of sales.

Encouraged to eat more

Portion size can influence intake as much as taste.
Prof. Brian Wansink
Cornell University

Large food packages and containers induce you into overeating, regardless of whether you like the food or not. This was the conclusion reached by Professor Brian Wansink of Cornell University and his researchers, following their investigation into whether environmental cues such as packaging and container size are so powerful that they can increase the intake of foods that are less palatable. Moviegoers were given stale popcorn that was two weeks old, in big buckets, and found that they ate 34% more than did those given the same stale popcorn in medium-sized containers. Moreover, if it tastes good then these figures rise even further. When served fresh popcorn in large tubs, people ate 45% more than those given fresh popcorn in medium-sized ones.

A further study in the Obesity Research publication by Prof. Wansink added further evidence to his research. He used a self-refilling soup bowl to examine whether what a person could see had any influence on the amount they ate and how full they felt. The experiment used participants, with differing ages and weight, who were placed in a restaurant style setting and were asked to eat a bowl of soup. Two types of soup bowls were used: 1. normal soup bowl, 2. a special self-refilling bowl, which very slowly and unnoticeably to the participant, added more soup. Participants who were unknowingly eating from self-refilling bowls ate 73% more than did those eating from the normal ones. Despite consuming a massive 73% more, they did not believe they had consumed more, or did they report feeling any fuller than did those eating from normal bowls.

These findings are consistent with the notion that the amount of food on a plate or bowl increases the amount of food a person will eat. It also showed that people will use visual markers, and not their feeling of fullness to determine how much to eat. Being visually influenced creates a situation where a person is likely to display reduced abilities to self-monitor the food they eat.

Although a large portion of McDonalds French fries is 147g per serving it does not 'visually' appear that large when compared, for example, to a jacket potato that is double its size at 300 grams. However, the fries pack 450 calories per serving and the jacket potato is only half that amount. Regardless of the calorie difference involved and any feelings of fullness, a person will eat the fries to excess; the larger the packaging or portion size the more a you will overeat; and the bigger the plates and bowls you use in your homes to serve foods on, the more food you are likely to eat.

The supermarkets and food manufacturers discourage you from purchasing small quantities of most foods and especially junk foods. There are greater price economies available in buying bigger packs for the consumer and bigger profits to be had for the food companies. Tie-in promotions positively encourage over consumption, for example, Pringles offering a free Blockbuster film for people purchasing three 200g packs (UK 2005). The food industry is in business to sell as much food and products as it can to return a healthy profit at year-end for its investors. Fruit and vegetables are inexpensive to buy but also make very little money for the supermarket. There is no supermarket in business today that has apples and pears at the checkout to tempt that last minute purchase.

Do you really have a choice?

> Since agriculture began, more than 7,000 species have been used as food or animal feed, and 30 crops now provide 95% of our food energy (wheat, rice, and maize alone provide more than 50%). Most of these plant[s] ... cannot survive in the wild and are maintained, literally, in farmers' fields, mainly in developing countries.
>
> *Food and Agriculture Organisation*
> *of the United Nations*

It needs to be repeated a few times in order to comprehend the fact that only 30 crops will provide 95% of the world foods.

When confronted with a supermarket superstore with endless isles and tens of thousands of products, is there an abundance of choice? Every year thousands of 'new' products are introduced to the marketplace. Will this increase your choice? There are over thirty different eye-catching packaged breakfast cereals for you to choose from, are their ingredients that different from each other?

There is a distinct lack of choice when, for example, you can only purchase three or four different varieties of apples year-round. As there are hundreds of different varieties of apples, you could be choosing from which are grown seasonally, and for most people, in locations closer than the ones which are imported onto the shelves of most supermarkets. Moving along the isles, of the over thirty different breakfast cereals on display you can buy, how many do not include wheat, corn, or rice in them, or do not contain the obligatory sugar as the second highest named ingredient, sprinkled with a questionable amount of salt?

For example, while shopping next time check out the top five ingredients of original Kellogg's Cornflakes. They will read something like this: milled corn, sugar, malt flavouring, high fructose corn syrup [sugar again], and salt. Your supermarket will have devoted one of the most frequented isles (towards the middle of the sales area) to the many different breakfast cereals; however, the apparent multiple choice is limited to just a handful of global companies who produce them. Kellogg's (United States) alone has a mind boggling fifty-eight different kinds of ready to eat cereals available to tempt you:

All-Bran® Bran Buds®, All-Bran® Extra Fiber, All-Bran® Original, All-Bran® Yogurt Bites, Apple Jacks®, Berry Krispies™, Caramel Nut Crunch™ , Cocoa Krispies™ , Complete® All-Bran® Oat Bran Flakes , Complete® All-Bran® Wheat Bran Flakes , Corn Pops® , Cracklin' Oat Bran® , Cran-Vanilla Crunch™ , Crispix® , Disney's Pirates of the Caribbean , Eggo™ Cereal Cinnamon Toast , Eggo™ Cereal Maple Syrup Froot Loops® , Froot Loops® 1/3 Less Sugar , Frosted Krispies® , Fruit Harvest™ Banana Berry , Fruit Harvest™ Peach Strawberry, Fruit Harvest™ Strawberry Blueberry , Honey Smacks® , Just Right® , Kellogg's Corn Flakes® , Kellogg's Frosted Flakes® , Kellogg's Frosted Flakes® 1/3 Less Sugar , Kellogg's Raisin Bran® , Kellogg's Smorz™ , Low Fat Granola With Raisins , Low Fat Granola without Raisins , Marshmallow Froot Loops™ , Mini Swirlz™ Cinnamon Bun , Mini-Swirlz™ Peanut Butter , Mini-Wheats® Frosted Bite Size , Mini-Wheats® Frosted Maple & Brown Sugar , Mini-Wheats® Frosted Original , Mini-Wheats® Frosted Strawberry Delight , Mini-Wheats® Frosted Vanilla Creme Bite Size , Mueslix® with Raisins, Dates & Almonds, Raisin Bran Crunch®, Rice Krispies® , Rice Krispies Treats® Cereal , Scooby-Doo!™ Berry Bones , Smart

Start® Antioxidants , Start® Healthy Heart, Smart Start® Healthy Heart Maple & Brown Sugar, Special K® , Special K® Fruit & Yogurt , Special K® Low Carb Lifestyle, Protein Plus , Special K® Red Berries , Special K® Vanilla Almond , Toasted Honey Crunch™ , Tony's Cinnamon Krunchers™, Organic Mini-Wheats® Frosted Bite Size , Organic Raisin Bran , Organic Rice Krispies®

Consumers will often site choice, as one of the factors in determining where they shop. Can it really be considered as consumer choice, when it is quite conceivable that a whole isle of the supermarket can display only cereals from one food giant? The picture starts to become a little clearer as you discover that despite the brightly coloured boxes and millions spent in advertising the 'different' products, the choice is limited to one or other of the food giants, just repackaged in a different way with virtually identical ingredients.

Barry Schwartz in his book 'The Paradox of Choice – Why Less is More', he demonstrates that people are overwhelmed with choice, and that having more choices are not necessarily a good thing. Highlighting consumer indecision as an issue, with the fact that consumers will on most occasions, make the wrong choices in order to 'just choose something' and move on. In his first chapter 'Let's Go Shopping', when conducting his initial investigations, he talks of finding 285 varieties of cookies in just one supermarket with chocolate chip cookies offering twenty-one different choices.

Curiosity catches the children

Children and adolescents are targeted aggressively by food advertisers using a wide range of marketing avenues and techniques to influence which products they buy.

- Over 70% of all food advertising is on TV
- About 40% of ads during children's programmes are for food
- Most ads are for confectionary, fast food, pre-sugared breakfast cereals, savoury snacks or soft drinks

Source: Food Standards Agency, UK

A study in the early nineties published in the Journal of the American Medical Association looked at brand advertising methods and their effects on children aged between three and six years, and revealed the strong similarities between the advertising and promotional methods used by food companies, and those of the tobacco industry, which were used to lure children into smoking.

The food, which is being touted to children, has been shown to be predominantly high in fat, sugar, and salt. Further studies provided increasing evidence that children exposed to food advertising, will prefer to choose advertised products, more frequently than the children not exposed to such adverts do. The more a child is exposed to the adverts the more they will request the product and the greater its availability in the home.

The global television company the BBC runs very successful programmes such as the Teletubbies and the Tweenies, to very young children. The characters on the programmes, with repeated viewing, are instantly recognisable by the children, and the BBC cashed in on this by allowing food companies to use this fact to sell their products successfully. The pictures of Teletubbies and Tweenies appeared on the packages of foods such as burgers and chips, custard cream biscuits, and crisps. The trouble is that young children who like the Teletubbies are too young to know that these foods are not very healthy. They just see the pictures on the packets, point to them in the supermarket, and 'ask' their parents to buy them. They probably do not even know what sort of food is in the packet before it is purchased.

The problem for the BBC arose when parents complained bitterly that the BBC should show some responsibility when granting the licences to companies allowing them to use the character images on their food products. The BBC were attacked from a different angle, when the Food Commission director, Tim Lobstein, stated that, 'For over two years we have urged the BBC to take children's health seriously when allowing their popular characters to be used to sell sweets, snacks, puddings and processed meals to children'.

In 2004 the BBC, after 'conducting its own research' eventually stopped allowing children's programme characters to be used on junk foods, and decided to use Teletubbies, Tweenies, and Fimbles characters only on 'healthy' foods. This was a victory for the health of children and some temporary respite for the parents!

As the problems of child obesity rage on, more and more governments look to tackle the advertisers and marketers who peddle the junk foods to them. The reactions of countries worldwide to this issue has been random and spread over decades. A report conducted by the World Health Organisation, 'Marketing Food to Children: the Global Regulatory Environment', reviewed the international practices in marketing of foods to children. Television remains the most popular means of promoting food and beverage worldwide, and even though 85% of the 73 countries reviewed, have some type of regulation in place relating to advertising to children, the global approach is incongruent, and in most countries useless.

European countries are a good example of the differing approaches; a couple of countries have total bans aimed at children under twelve. Others have regulations in pace aimed at restricting advertising to children: adverts before and after children's programmmes prohibited; advertising toys between 7am and 11am not allowed; adverts during cartoons prohibited; direct product advertising of goods not allowed; cartoon character sales pitches prohibited; children's television personalities cannot advertise any products before 9pm. The list of differentiating regulations goes on from country to country and continent to continent, and the World Health Organisation report leaves a sting in the tail; 'it is not clear how these regulations are applied, interpreted and enforced.' Using the example that satellite television channels are not regulated in what adverts they can show to children.

Banning junk food advertising aimed at children, as is the case in Norway and Sweden (ban in place since the early nineties), and the Canadian province Quebec (since 1980), has not been shown to solve the problem of child obesity. The incongruent global approach may attract a small portion of the blame for this failure but the major blame continues to be aimed at the food giants' ability to stay one-step ahead of the slow moving wheels of government, which can be viewed as the major cause of the continued rise in the risks of your child becoming obese.

- Companies spent an estimated $10 billion in 2004 marketing food and beverages to children.
- About one-third of children's daily calories come from food consumed outside of the home.
- Children aged two to fifteen influences the purchase of about $500 billion worth of food and beverages a year.

SOURCE: Institute of Medicine
National Academic Press

A total ban on television junk food advertising to children will not solve the problem, as there are always new ways available in which the food companies can carry on with business as usual. The techniques used include the use of school activities, product placement in children's shows and programmes or popular films, induce impulse purchases, link food to sport (and famous sportspeople), target advertising, sponsoring events and clubs, co-marketing with toys, books, clothes, etc., competitions and promotions, the internet, games, and mobile phone adverts. Children are now exposed from a very early age to a wide variety of advertisers and marketers in various media forms. These messages come from all angles and available almost everywhere you go: from your home, to schools, child care facilities, supermarkets, shopping centres, cinemas, sports events, restaurants, special calendar occasions, and the waiting rooms of doctors and dentists.

Branded toys are just one example, which help create and feed a child's familiarity of the brand colours and shapes, and can influence their present and future purchase preferences, which can give rise to either parent-pester-power purchases (when they cannot buy it for themselves) or 'triggered' solo purchases (when they have the cash to buy it). You can buy almost any branded food or drink children's toy or game.

> **The list goes on and on with items such as:**
> OREO Barbie doll; The OREO, Kellogg's Pizza Hut, M&M, Coca Cola, and Snickers sponsored racing cars; McDonald's Play Restaurant Set, Cheerios Counting Book; The Coca Cola branded: Classic Ads Monopoly, Super Size Domino game, and 500-piece puzzle. The M&M's branded: Brand Chocolate Candies Counting Board Book, Brand Counting Book, Brand Chocolate Candies Math, Brand Count to One Hundred Book, Brand Color Pattern Book, Brand Birthday Book, Brand Easter Egg Hunt, All-American Parade Book, Halloween Treat Book, Brand Valentine Book, Thanksgiving Feast, and Christmas Gift Book. Kellogg's Froot Loops! Counting Fun Book; Kellogg's Froot Loops! Color Fun Book; Coca Cola Checkers; Coca Cola Playing cards
>
> *Source:Amazon.com*

If at first they do not succeed

Children do not have the defences, or proficiency, to discriminate from commercial or non-commercial content, or able to identify the persuasive elements of advertising, and more importantly, they cannot do it without being asked explicitly to do so. As a result, children are confronted with techniques, which are specifically created to implant lasting images of manufacturer's products into their innocent lives; these implanted images will influence preference, purchase, and future loyalty of products.

School activities and supplies

Supplies offered to schools such as free books or sports equipment linked to token collections, which also increases consumption of products such as breakfast cereals, chocolate, and crisps.

Product placement in children's shows and programmes or popular films

M&M's brand confectionery unveiled its white chocolate limited edition range, which includes White Chocolate Pirate Pearls confectionery with the United States release of the movie 'Pirates of the Caribbean: Dead

Man's Chest'. The food giant Burger King collaborates with DreamWorks and Nickelodeon for co-branding, and McDonald's Corporation has a contract with Disney.

Induce impulse purchases
Sell new products at a low price or with multiple buy incentives, to encourage you to try them or buy more. Use big bold colours to tempt you into the store. Place junk food displays in areas of maximum usage to attract maximum attention and purchase. Use multiple display stands and posters around the store to keep trying to get that 'impulse' buy. Moreover, do not forget the displays of snacks near the checkout where children and parents arrive, in a bored and stressed state, triggering that impulse (or pestered) purchase.

Link food to sport (and famous sportspeople)
Another way to by-pass regulations on advertising food and beverage manufacturers have become highly competitive to capture the youth market, and youth appeal is being built into advertising targeted to broader audiences and specifically to adolescents. Celebrity endorsements such as footballers David Beckham (Pepsi and Coca-Cola) & Ronaldinho (Pepsi); music celebrities Christina Aguilera (Coca Cola), Madonna (Pepsi), Beyonce (Pepsi) , Shakira (Pepsi) links a brand to a fan base and are designed to appeal to all.

Co-marketing with toys, books, clothes, etc
United States fast food giant McDonald's has a range of children's clothing. The McKids range which is designed and made in China, with a line of products, which include toys, videos, DVDs, and books.

The Internet
Children under eighteen years old, represent around 20% of those using the internet, and here you can find some of the new approaches to children. Every page they surf on the internet gives advertisers and companies clues to what children like. This information is used to build a 'consumer' profile and then put to work when 'targeting' children with tailored advertisements. Competitions and promotions lure them into other websites, joining mailing lists or providing personal details, which are always used. Website games, commonly referred to as 'advergames', are interactive and draw the user in to spend more time on the website, to buy a product, or to simply increase product awareness. Other forms of subtle persuasion include games, which have advertising within a game, similar to product placement advertising in films, where the advertising content is within the movie or game 'world'. For example, it may be a sports simulation, which carries real product 'adverts' representing major

corporations, such as Nike, Adidas, McDonalds, Burger King, Nokia, Ericsson, and Sony.

Children prompted to advertise to their friends

Viral marketing, as its name suggests, seeks to spread commercial messages in the same way that a virus spreads from one individual to another. Viral commercials take the shape of funny video clips, interactive games, images or jokes which children will find entertaining enough to pass on to their friends.

Mobile phone adverts

It is estimated that nine out of ten children under the age of sixteen now own a mobile phone. Junk food companies have used the mobile phone to run competitions encouraging children to supply their mobile phone numbers and other details. Promotional codes printed on food or drink packaging are requested to be texted in to the companies in exchange for prizes. Once the food company has your number, they use it to advertise new offers and induce you to buy more products or services.

Food labels

Are food labels misleading; deceiving; confusing; incorrect; and fraudulent? In an article published in a recent issue of the American Journal of Preventive Medicine, researchers undertook a cross-sectional study from June 2004 to April 2005, with a wide socioeconomic range. Each participant was required to complete a Nutrition Label Survey, designed with input from professionals such as registered dieticians and primary care physicians. The survey results showed that people find it hard to decipher and understand the nutritional information or health claims on food packaging labels.

Further research published in the Journal of Consumer Affairs provided details of a controlled experiment, which examined the effectiveness of various front-sided health claims when used in combination with a full health claim on the back of a package. The results indicate that combining short health claims on the front of a package with full health claims on the back leads consumers to believe and act on the claim. Manufacturers may make statements such as 'builds strong bones,' 'strengthens memory,' 'relieves stress,' 'increases energy,' 'improves sleep,' and these type messages to influence a 'healthy' purchase. There is more to strong bones than just eating a calcium-rich food, and more to human memory, stress, energy, or sleep than the isolating and eating a beneficial food nutrient.

These messages are more confusing than helpful, worthless to the consumer, and may provide a false impression of the health value of the food product. It is not surprising then, when some of these food labels and health claims are misleading the consumer into thinking food products have health benefits, or have healthier ingredients when they do not. Food companies take advantage of loopholes and lax food labelling regulations to promote and advertise their products using these 'health' claims.

Food labels should help the consumer make an intelligent decision about the safety of the product and its nutritional value. Unfortunately, this is not always the case. There are no internationally recognised nutritional labelling laws, with different countries adopting differing laws and widely differing enforcement policies. Until countries and governments look to harmonise the food labelling laws the consumer will be at a greater risk of being misled by advertisers and marketers. The food industry has firmly opposed any plans to modify existing food labels with representatives claiming that 'there are no bad products, and the problems come from bad eating habits'. Moreover, they can be found frequently flexing their lobbying powers to influence food laws, which could disrupt their huge profits.

In a recent example, The European Parliament and the European Union's member states, under pressure from the food industry, had to compromise proposed legislation which would have seen food products which use tags like 'high fibre,' 'light' or 'vitamin rich' only be allowed on foods which were also not high in fat, sugar, or salt. The new compromised law in effect sends out a confusing and conflicting message; it will continue to allow food companies to market and advertise food products such as lollipops as 'fat free' implying a healthy food, even though the majority of the product is simple sugar, which is positively unhealthy. It leaves the loophole wide open for food companies to continue to exploit and influence unhealthy food purchases.

The deceptive and distractive headlines featured prominently on food packaging should be blatantly ignored; opting instead for a quick scan of the ingredients listing. For example, labels that state 'fat-free' should be immediately suspected; and viewed with scepticism. The clever marketing tricksters have mastered the art of selling to the 'fat' fearing consumers. You should be aware that any reduced fat or fat-free claim means very little until you have read the small print. As a product that is, 97% fat free can still contain around 30% fat; and remember, it is not just the content of fat, which you have to be aware of, but it is more important to be aware of what types of fat are present within that food.

A marketing trick
Firstly, the advertisers claim will use the weight of the product to calculate the percentages and not the calories. For instance, 97% fat-free

contains 3% fat in weight terms, which equates to 3 grams of fat per 100g of the product. Fat represents nine kcal of energy per gram, therefore, the total fat calories for the product will be, a not so fat-free, 27% per 100g. Milk is another example of the marketing tricks you have lived with for decades. Whole milk derives more than half of its calories from fat and even the excessively hyped skimmed milk secures 38% of its calories from it.

All health claims should be viewed with a positive scepticism and foods containing 'no cholesterol' are no exception, as you may be distracted from the real menace in the foods. For example, no vegetable fats contain cholesterol. Therefore, foods can perfectly legally be labelled as cholesterol-free, and mask the fact that the frequently used vegetable fats such as coconut, palm, and palm kernel oil are very high in saturated fats. This cholesterol-free mask will hide the fact that saturated fats are seen as 'cholesterol producers' once inside the body.

Often a product may be labelled with useless headline grabbing words such as 'lite,' 'light,' or 'diet,' and as they carry no legal definition, are useless indicators to the healthiness of the food product.

The way forward
Instead of listing the hundreds of items, you need to watch out for on the ingredients list, this has been kept super-simple and you only have one guideline you should follow:

- **Choose food products that list less than *five* ingredients on the label**

Supermarket selling bad apples
Supermarkets are cornering the market; adding to global pollution, encouraging bad food production practices and driving local producers and retailers out of business; flooding the shop floor with an average of 20,000 food items in its superstores, which corresponds to a less than 1% choice of which can be considered 'real' food. Consumers are constantly being oversold to, and offered value promotions (such as buy-one-get-one-free, 3 for the price of 2, and artificially discounted prices) on foods and drinks, which are mostly negatively correlated to your continued health and wellness.

In a report conducted by the National Consumer Council (NCC), the leading British supermarket chains are strongly criticised for their low-cost or economy-range foods, which the report claims are much less healthy than their more expensive counterparts. Most low cost lines on offer, which are predominantly purchased by the less affluent consumers such as the young and elderly, contained significantly more salt, slightly more fat and sugar than the supermarkets own-brand counterparts. In addition, it was shown that there are fewer healthy food promotions in supermarkets where poorer consumers are likely to shop. Of the 94 standard products the NCC surveyed, 41 (44%) met the Food Standards Agency's new sodium target level for 2006, based on acceptable healthy limits. Of the 49 economy products surveyed only 17 (35%) met the target.

Lord Whitty, chairperson of the NCC, said of the findings: 'Consumers who rely heavily on economy ranges are clearly being short-changed on health. Supermarkets poor performance on economy lines is a backward step since last year. At least 26 million people are eating too much salt - most of it hidden in the food we buy - and supermarkets should play a bigger part in tackling the problem.' He added that, 'Supermarkets have made progress on reducing salt in their standard food lines, so there's no good reason why they can't do the same with economy lines. Supermarkets should behave more responsibly. Budget-conscious shoppers must not be shut out from eating healthily.'

Danger: Health barriers

Your nourishment is no longer a simple and direct process from farm to fork. Instead, internal and external pressures, often in unison, influence your daily living and cause major disruptions to you and your health. You need to keep your eyes open and your wits about you in order to live healthily.

Supermarkets taking over the world

Tesco now controls 30% of the grocery market in the UK. In 2006, the supermarket chain announced over £2.2 billion in profits. Growing evidence indicates that Tesco's success is partly based on trading practices that have serious consequences for suppliers, farmers and workers worldwide, local shops and the environment. Moreover, the growth is not limited to the UK, with Tesco operating in twelve different international markets, serving over 15 million people, and raking in £7.6bn in sales.

And Tesco just one of the fish in an ever decreasing sea; with other global giants like the United States giant Wal-Mart, the French Carrefour, the Dutch multinational Ahold, striving to monopolise the food retailing industry at the expense of your health.

The politics of food

The force the food industry can affect on governments is immense and the results are most often at a detriment to your health. Mountains of food lie in wait in stockrooms, warehouses, and storage depots while the profit hungry food industry just continue to produce, persuade, and sell its products to a growing (literally) consumer.

Marion Nestle, a professor at the New York University, wrote an exposé on the behind the scenes food industry. The book, Food Politics, not surprisingly created a storm of controversy. Nestle was the editor of the 1988 Surgeon General's Report on Nutrition and Health, therefore is uniquely qualified to cut through the maze of food industry interests and influences. She vividly illustrates food politics in action, with examples of watered-down government dietary advice, and the 'pushing' of diet supplements.

Economics and politics drive the mass production and consumption of food, with the health and well-being of the consumer trailing a few billion dollars of profit behind. People will struggle to find untainted advice on what to eat and how to stay healthy. Governments are pushed and pulled by the lobbying of the food industry ensuring business as usual. Nutritional experts are 'guided' into towing the government line (of the day), while the food industry flexes it financial muscle outside of the political arena when threatened by such exposés, such as Marion Nestle's Food Politics. They can call upon their vast manpower resources to 'bad mouth' or 'talk up' products and services for economic gain (a good example can always be found on the website amazon.com, where 'disguised' industry representatives will 'bad mouth' any book which may dissuade consumers from buying or asking awkward questions about products – classic propaganda).

The food industry pressure has resulted in a massive campaign to divert public opinion away from the food industry and firmly onto the consumer. Governments chose the route of non-confrontation with the food industry, and put the blame of all the overweight and obesity epidemics on the lack of physical activity. It is the non-controversial route, as everyone can agree on the fact that increasing physical activity is of benefit to health. However, governments fail miserably and repeatedly, as they continue to ignore nutritional problems, which have the effect of rendering physical activity impotent.

Experts here, there, and everywhere
Experts who have allegiances and financial arrangements, which amount to conflict of interest, continue to infiltrate communication pathways (television, radio, magazines, newspapers, etc.) and take prominent advice-wielding positions in public life. This trend was picked up in the article, 'Food company sponsorship of nutrition research and professional activities: a conflict of interest?' in which many examples showed the extent of the expert bias. Over 30% of university and research faculties, where much of the health information originates, accepted industry funding. In a more blatant conflict of interests, nutritional fact sheets issued by the American Dietetic Association,

included sponsors such as NutraSweet, Mars, Nabisco, and Campbell Soup, leading to tainted advice.

For instance, look below at the heavily influenced advice given in the nutritional fact sheets issued by the American Dietetic Association.

> **NutraSweet (producers of artificial sweeteners) on Aspartame**:
> 'Aspartame makes available a wide variety of food and beverage choices for the person interested in maintaining a healthful lifestyle'
>
> **Mars (leading chocolate snack producer) on Chocolate**:
> 'Chocolate is no longer a concern for those wary of saturated fat, and in fact, chocolate can be part of a heart-healthy eating plan'
>
> **Nabisco (producers of cookie like the Oreo's) on Snacking**:
> 'In today's busy world, snacking is part of our daily routine. We enjoy milk and cookies after school and reach for a handful of crackers before bed'
>
> **Campbell Soup (producers of sodium containing soups) on Sodium**:
> 'The link between the sodium you eat and high blood pressure is unclear'

Glamorising unhealthy behaviour

Diet and cookbooks in most instances, glamorise unhealthy behaviours, and not surprisingly are continually in the bestsellers lists. The irony is that as one helps you lose weight, the other helps you to regain any weight you may have lost. The diet books gather evidence to prove that their slimming program is the best way to lose weight, and attack and chastise what you eat presently, and seek to instil restrictions according to their theories of what is causing your overweight state. On the other hand, the cookbooks and their entourage of celebrity chefs, and media all systematically glamorise food, its preparation, its many must-have cooking utensils, must-use condiments, endless variations of global recipes, and meal course combinations, leading to regular wastage and over consumption. To make matters worse, after a person discontinues a diet (which everyone eventually does), their body weight will usually go beyond their pre-diet weight.

All cooking programmes, cookbooks, restaurants, and providers of food, should have to provide nutritional information on all the products they promote or supply. This would give the consumer all the relevant information necessary to make a choice relevant to their health circumstances and empower a proactive decision-making process, as oppose to one of guesswork.

The supplement sting
Alternative treatments and dietary supplements are multi billion dollar industries and mostly play on the fears of suffers looking for a quick fix to their ailment or nutritional inefficiencies. Marketing ploys draw upon consumer insecurities and misinformation with claims that are often too good to be true, lack proven medical research, and too simplistic in its diagnosis and treatment. Alternative treatments are designed to appeal to anyone, but certain conditions and populations are more likely to be targeted. The vulnerable will find it difficult to refuse a miracle cure in the face of their suffering, and be unable to question things critically. Conditions can range from aging to arthritis, and cancer to AIDS, with most treatments available offering very little change in the daily living for users.

Dietary supplements for most healthy adults are an unnecessary expense (refer to Vitamins & Minerals section in Nourishment). Tapping into fears of vitamin and mineral deficiencies and their associated diseases, the supplement industry promotes numerous kinds of solutions in many different guises. The more vulnerable are more at risk of turning to products such as the high-potency supplement, which of course can be harmful and toxic to the body if abused. For most people a one-a-day multivitamin and mineral supplement that meets 100% of the recommended daily intake for each vitamin and some minerals is more than adequate.

The weight loss charade
Your choices of fad diets, drugs, special foods, and health services are countless; not to mention self-help books, DVD's, seminars, classes, programs, and all the media productions from television to radio. All sell the dream of weight-loss in the fastest and most convenient way. If there were one that actually worked and provided a long-term solution for overweight and obese people, then you would ALL know about it. It is with great regret however to note that there is no 'miracle' solution out there, and in fact in some cases the products or services available are dangerous and harmful.

The diet industry is cashing in, while they sell you the next fad or fashion food or diet. The irony is that the same global companies which supply the foods which been linked to overweight and obesity factors such as, foods which are high in sugar, salt, fat, and 'empty' calories, are also the same companies which own the 'health and diet' food ones. The result is a perfect win-win scenario for the global food giants as first they make money by 'fattening' you up, and then the make even more money by trying to 'slim' you down.

Read all about it (again, and again, and again)
There is not a day, which goes by without an item of news that does not claim a new breakthrough in human health and wellness. The problem is there is so much information available that finding the appropriate news that is both relevant to your lifestyle or takes into consideration your other health factors is like landing a winning lottery ticket. Pressure to conform to the latest research is magnified by the media, as the news-hungry agencies clamour over themselves to locate the next big thing. You only need to pick up your weekend newspaper to find out which is the current food fashion destined to heal all your ailments or which is the miracle diet slicing off the weight.

The old adage of 'don't believe everything your read in the newspapers' can be said for all the forms of old and new media. Especially as no person can truly follow all the 'advice' given and expect to experience positive change in their health.

Part four

R & R

R&R for some might mean 'rest' and 'relaxation' while for the Health-Warrior it stands for something a whole lot more; Repair & Rejuvenation. The attitudes of people are continually being manipulated, and in this modern world are influenced from multiple directions making it hard to focus on the ideal path. The following chapters will identify the problems, and provide the solutions on how to stay calm while under constant attack.

How can you keep a level head when others are losing theirs? Where do you find the inner-strength to improve lifestyle choices and develop wellness-inspiring habits? Can you empower yourself mentally, and protect yourself from irrelevant, unhelpful, and harmful distractions?

After, the air you breathe, the water you drink, and the food you eat, the next most important factor contributing to your quality of life (and survival), is sleep and there is no substitute for it. Good health demands good sleep, and there is a lot more to it than just putting your feet up or grabbing forty winks. The chapters that follow, will look at the process of sleep, and the problems caused by a lack of it, and provide tried and tested formulas to maximise it.

'Relax-tivity' is one such solution and is derived from the words 'relaxation' and 'activity'; and is something that you can adapt to your personal circumstances to assist the repair and rejuvenation of your body. As mentioned above and worth reiterating, there is no substitute for an uninterrupted nights sleep. However, used in conjunction with the appropriate amount of good quality sleep, Relax-tivity will encompass outstanding mind and body benefiting activities. It includes activities such as breathing and meditative activities, physical activity, positive thinking, radiant people, visualisation, self-massage, music, smell, and the natural environment, to establish 'my essential time-out' (MeTo) opportunities for you to use at will to create an atmosphere for your continued health and well-being.

Chapter 12

The Mark of the Zzzz's

Good health demands good sleep and the importance it carries can be drawn from the fact that you will spend around one third of your life asleep. The exact reasons as to why sleep is needed still confound the scientists of today as they did of yesteryears. Sleep maintains your circadian rhythms, the light-dependent 24-hour cycle that regulates your body and mind. With optimum sleep the body and mind will be rested, repaired, reset, and readied for the day ahead; and you can expect to experience better quality of life, improved performance, a boosted immune system, slow the aging process, and harbour a stronger physical and mental disposition (opening the way for increased memory, learning, and concentration).

> The beginning of health is sleep.
> *Irish Proverb*

Just some of the benefits of a good night of quality sleep:

- increased alertness
- cheerful
- optimum memory, learning, and concentration
- maximum energy and creativity

A lack of sleep, in recent studies, has been associated with increased levels of obesity, gastrointestinal illnesses, increased risks of heart and cardiovascular diseases, diabetes, chronic fatigue, weakened immune system (leading to increased frequencies of illnesses such as colds and flu), increased risk of accidents, and mental illnesses such as depression and anxiety.

People are sleeping on average less than a generation ago. They are suffering activity and sensory overload from the modern world, and are subsequently failing to claim the quality sleep that good health demands.

O, Somnus,
divine repose of all things!
Gentlest of the deities!
Peace to the troubled mind,
from which you drive the cares of life.
Restorer of men's strength
when wearied with the toils of day.

Ovid, Metamorphoses
Book XI (1 AD)

How much sleep is enough?

There is no one number, which fits all, as sleep requirements will depend on factors such as environment, stress, health, gender, and age. Your sleep architecture will change with your age; a baby will sleep the most, which can be as much as twenty hours in the day, and from there on it reduces on a sliding scale through childhood, adolescence, adults, to older adults who may be grateful for a few hours sleep. The consensus is that adults function best with between seven to nine hours of uninterrupted sleep.

What happens when you sleep?

When you sleep, your body will experience reduced movement and a decreased awareness of your surroundings, though this awareness can be easily interrupted by external stimulation, such as a loud noise. Most animals enjoy the benefits of sleep, with total amounts of sleep differing from species to species. Most of them will close their eyes and adopt particular sleep postures when sleeping. Scientists have been able to track brain activities while a person is asleep by using a procedure called electroencephalography (EEG). With this kind of evaluation of brain activity, and similar procedures for the body and eye, they were able to explore the different sections during sleep.

Rapid eye movement (REM) was coined by the American physiologists Eugene Aserinsky and Nathaniel Kleitman in the 1950's, when subjects in their experiments experienced periods of eye twitching during sleep. Further studies showed that when the subjects were awakened during REM sleep they reported vivid dreams. REM sleep has been shown to be most like the times a person is awake, because brain wave activity is short and rapid just like the brain activity of a wakeful state.

Non rapid eye movement (NREM) is simply that; a time in the sleep cycle when a person will experience little or no eye movement.

This sleep stage is characterised by physiological changes such as breathing and heart rate slows down; body temperature and blood pressure tend to decrease; and subjects awakened during NREM are less likely to report vivid, action packed dreams. The brain wave activity is, in contrast to the short and rapid movements of REM sleep, larger and slower.

Sleep studies have shown that humans will move between REM and NREM sleep in regular patterns. The average person will experience the vivid and film-like dreams of REM sleep about every 90 minutes. These REM moments will tend to last from ten minutes, for those experienced at the beginning of sleep, to thirty minutes experienced in the hours just before you awake. About twenty percent of your sleep time will be spent in REM sleep. Before entering REM sleep, you will go through stages of NREM sleep. These stages of NREM sleep will last 90 minutes and in this time, you will gradually fall into deeper levels of sleep, experiencing slower breathing and heart rates, and decreased body temperature and blood pressure. Once you have achieved the deepest stage of NREM sleep you will slowly ascend back through the levels until you progress into REM sleep. In a normal nights sleep you can experience up to six cycles of REM sleep.

The brain and sleep
The brain plays a major role in how and when a person sleeps. The brainstem the portion of the brain just above the spinal cord is critical in REM sleep control, while the forebrain is important in NREM sleep. Some parts of the brain are only active during REM sleep while others are completely inactive. The brain neurons responsible for REM sleep also control the muscle tone of your body during this time; most muscles (except for eye and breathing muscles) will be relaxed. The major muscle groups such as the back, neck, arms, and legs will be relaxed during REM sleep, which goes some way to explain why you do not act out your vivid dreams while sleeping.

The forebrain area is where the most neural activity will take place before and during NREM sleep. Most of these neurons are activated by heat, and is the reason why you will enjoy a good night's sleep after a warm bath, spend time in an over-heated room, on a sunny day, or at the beach or park.

Even though it seems the brain is in constant use twenty-four hours a day, leading scientists are starting to believe that the brain is actually rested, reset, and rejuvenated during sleep. REM sleep can be looked at as the time for 'brain housework'; a time to put things back in the places they should be, get rid of useless items, collate and batch things so it's easier to find later, and clear the way for new things. While

NREM sleep is more like journey to the car mechanic, where you are physically repaired and restored ready for the next day.

Tick-tock
Located in the hypothalamus, the circadian clock has been shown to be, in addition to being the principle source of virtually all your physiological processes, a key player in the synchronising of sleep and wake behaviours. In other words, it can ultimately make you feel sleepy at one end of your sleep cycle, alert and awake at the opposite end. Your circadian clock, despite any moves by society to operate twenty-four hours a day, exerts a strict control on times of sleep and wakefulness. This conflict between the circadian clock (the natural synergy between the body needs and environment), and modern life patterns can be plainly viewed when you experience problems such as jet-lag, night and shift-work sleeping disorders, and sleeping pattern changes you experience between the summer and winter seasons. Most people will find it easier to get out of bed earlier on a summers day when it is brighter, warmer, and alive to the sounds of birds etc., as oppose to a cold and dark winters day regardless of the time they usually awake.

> And We made your sleep as a thing for rest.
>
> *The Noble Qur'an*
> *Surat An-Naba' (The News)*

Guaranteed sleep tips to get optimum sleep time and quality

- **Establish a sleep routine**; make it clear to your body and mind that it is sleep time. Perform similar rituals before each nights sleep. Activities such as listening to the same calming music, cleansing your body, and brushing your teeth at similar times each night, reading an unchallenging book, or random page-filling writing, if used regularly will help establish a sleep routine.
- **Avoid overheating** the bedroom (lose the electric blankets and turn off the central heating at night). Even during cold winter nights, your choice should be to wear extra bedclothes as oppose to using other heating sources.
- **If possible, sleep with windows open** or try to ensure a pathway for the circulation of air through your bedroom.
- **Your place of sleep should be clutter-free**, painted in neutral colours, cleaned regularly (with sheeting frequently aired) and be free of any electrical appliances (especially the TV).
- **Avoid exposure to bright lighting** in the evening hours (and wear an eye mask to bed if light sensitive); Dimmed lights at night will

help promote the secretion of melatonin, a hormone that is produced by the brain to help regulate your sleepiness.

- **Avoid anger and negative emotional situations** (or at least, make peace before sleep).
- **Maintain similar sleep and wake times** throughout the week and weekend.
- **Cleanse the body**; a clean body will help you sleep better.
- **Physical activity during the day or night** helps you fall asleep quicker (and will not hinder your sleep).
- **Cleanse the mind**; leave the stresses and strains of the day outside the bedroom.
- **Actively seek to get at least 20 minutes of morning sun** or day light as early as is possible.
- **Listen to your body;** if it is not ready for sleep then do something sleep inducing until your body and mind are ready (see Relax-tivity).
- **Practice Relax-tivity** (see Chapter 14 - Relax-tivity & MeTo opportunities).
- **Eat foods, which can help you, sleep**: such as bananas, figs, chicken, tuna, turkey, milk, yoghurt, sunflower seeds, almonds, hazelnuts, green vegetables, and whole grains.
- **Avoid foods that disturb your sleep**: excess sugar, highly refined products, fatty foods, and individual foods such as pork, cheese, chocolate, aubergines, tomatoes, and potatoes.
- **Avoid all stimulants** (such as caffeine, alcohol, and smoking) especially in the evening; this will raise the cortisol levels in your body, which keep you awake.
- **Avoid large volumes of food or drink** within two hours of sleep time; indigestion and having to get up to use the bathroom will reduce the quality of your sleep; go for healthy sleep-inducing snacks instead.
- **Avoid junk television** including violent, dramatic programmes and films.
- **Avoid napping**; it will inhibit your sleeping patterns and only offer questionable benefits; you should practice Relax-tivity instead.
- **Avoid sleeping pills**, medicines, dietary supplements (such as melatonin) and other unnatural sleeping aids, as your quality of sleep will be subsequently reduced.

Chapter 13

Don't snooze & you lose

Your sleep is a supremely effective process, which is orchestrated by intricate networks and transmitters in your brain. Sleep is easily interrupted by internal and external factors, which in turn can lead to malfunctions in your body. A lack of sleep has become an overlooked danger and damaging problem, costing billions to the health service. Modern living conditions are promoting more sleepless nights with familiar and persistent problems, such as lethargy (even after a nights sleep), difficulty in getting to sleep, interrupted sleep, and the inability to sleep after being awakened.

> Sleep serves to cool the brain
>
> *Aristotle*

In recent studies, it has been shown that with, at least 70% of adolescents suffering from mild to severe sleep depravation, and 50% of adults and over 68% of older adults reporting one or more sleep problems, the signs are ominous for human health and continued well-being. People will respond to sleep loss in similar ways; when REM sleep loss occurs, it is made up for by a spending longer and more intense period in REM sleep at the next sleep opportunity. The same can be said of NREM sleep loss, as any loss will be made up for, in a longer and deeper NREM sleep. This proves that you require both forms of sleep to function at your optimum capacity, and conversely proves that any shortfall in either sleep forms will lead to a detrimental effect on your physiological functions and physical and mental well-being.

A period of lost sleep carries an exponentially larger debt to pay; at the minimal level, sleep loss will cause a reduction an alertness and attentiveness, with increases in mood swings and irritability. Your ability to perform the simplest tasks will suffer and this lack of concentration and judgement will lead to increases in accidents (car and workplace).

In a recent 12-year study, researchers confirmed the worrying links between sleeping problems and serious diseases. It was shown that people who slept less than five hours per night, and had difficulty in maintaining sleep, had an increase prevalence of diabetes.

Longer term sleep loss can lead to obesity, gastrointestinal illnesses, increased risks of heart and cardiovascular diseases, diabetes, chronic fatigue, weakened immune system (leading to more frequent illnesses such as colds and flu), and mental illnesses such as depression and anxiety. According to Tim Steury at the Washington State University, USA, periods without sleep will have progressively dramatic effects on well-being. The downward spiral starts with a reduction in attention and learning abilities.

Further sleep deprivation will increase the speed of your body engine (the metabolic rate), and adversely affect your ability to control body temperature. As sleep denial continues, it will lead to hallucinations, and ultimately death (though there is no recorded research in humans to prove this final step, in has been shown to be the case in sleep-deprived rats).

Children, adolescents, and sleep
The problems of lack of sleep are important for all, but are especially important for those still developing their physical, mental, emotional, and cognitive functions, such as children and adolescents. To secure a brighter future for your children, then you have to take a proactive role in their health and wellness.

It is commonplace for children to demand, at get a television for their bedroom, and this trend is growing in number and is occurring at a younger age. It is disturbing then to review recent studies, in which researchers looking at the sleeping habits of children concluded that television viewing clearly disturbed the amount of quality sleep they received. Children younger than three years old who viewed television were shown to display irregular sleep patterns, and the evening viewing of television for schoolchildren was associated with at least one type of sleep disturbance.

As the age of the children increased so did the prevalence of their sleep problems. In a recent study looking at over 3,000 adolescents, it was shown that 70% of them experienced mild to severe sleep depravation, and this was shown to have an adverse effect on their studies. Furthermore, if these adolescents are not given adequate amounts of sleep, of not less than six to eight hours, then you can expect to see an increase in their health problems. A study specifically investigating this problem, identified that the lack of adequate sleep was shown to reduce the life appreciation of the adolescents, their responsibility for good health (being less likely to adopt a good diet), and were less likely to manage their stress levels. Whereas, adequate amounts of sleep (of more than six to eight hours) were associated with lower levels of obesity, reduced visits to the doctor, and positive behaviour.

In college students, the lack of sleep was identified as a major factor leading to depression, at two times more common than in the general population.

Sleep disorders

The most common sleep disorder is insomnia; this is where a previously good sleeper suffers from chronic sleep loss over a period of weeks or longer. True chronic insomnia is still relatively rare, though you would not believe it if you look at the amount of drugs (both prescription and over-the-counter) in daily use. The highly addictive sleep-inducing drugs were only designed for short-term use, as a chronic sleep disorder is a sign of a more serious underlying problem such as chronic anxiety, depression, stress, use of other drugs, and stimulants, and imbalances in body chemistry.

If you experience any of the following symptoms over a period of weeks, you should seek further professional advice to establish the root of the problem:

- Have trouble getting to sleep
- Wake up frequently during the night
- Fall asleep at inappropriate times even after a night of sleep
- Have sudden energy slumps or bouts of uncontrollable sleep
- Have nightmares (you cannot recollect) that interrupt your sleep
- Experience morning (not drink related) hangovers and headaches often

Say no to sleeping drugs

As with most drug interventions to 'treat' human ailments, you are confronted with ominous problems and changes in physiological functions. For instance, sleeping pills and anti-depressants can change the way the brain functions in their enthusiasm to get you to sleep, and suppresses and reduces your amount of REM sleep. This in turn, will reduce the 'brain housework' necessary for your mental well-being, and it will increase your stress-response reducing your sleep duration. Further reducing the time, you spend in REM sleep. This is a dangerous vicious circle.

The sleeping pills come in many forms from Valium to Librium, from Ativan to Zanax, and all have something else very much in common. They are all highly addictive and have very powerful side effects, and should be avoided at all costs. The side effects, not only create nervousness, confusion, irritability, aggressiveness, hallucinations, and out of character behaviour for the user, but can include other effects such as:

<table>
<tr><td>Impaired brain functions: memory</td><td>Diarrhoea</td></tr>
<tr><td>Suppression of REM sleep</td><td>Depression</td></tr>
<tr><td>Drowsiness</td><td>Dizziness</td></tr>
<tr><td>Dizziness</td><td>Impaired co-ordination</td></tr>
<tr><td>Morning hangovers</td><td>Indigestion</td></tr>
<tr><td>Nausea</td><td>Constipation</td></tr>
<tr><td>Lethargy</td><td>Blurred vision</td></tr>
</table>

Working and sleep

Society no longer seems to enjoy the benefits of the days when there were clear distinctions between working times and social ones; those borders are now flexible and interspersed. The 24/7 (twenty-four hours a day / seven days a week) society has embraced shift work, night work, irregular, and flexible working hours to accommodate the 'demands' of business and the consumer; leading to the availability of the majority of products and services day and night.

Newer technologies (like the Internet and multifunctional mobile phones) facilitate this drive to a 24/7 society built on the demands of business and the consumer, who have ever expanding reach, in a truly global marketplace. For employers, company boardrooms, and shareholders this ticks all the right boxes and is looked on with the most favourable eyes. In a recent study which conducted an in-depth review retracing over thirty-eight years (1966-2004) of research, looking specifically at the sleeping problems of shift-work employees and its effects on the workplace, and the health of the employees, found that in most cases the employees experienced detrimental effects. The effects included increased absenteeism and sick leave, reduced efficiency, a poor physical and psychological health status; and when compared to non-shift-work employees were shown to have increased risks of hypertension, obesity, lipid (fat) abnormalities, diabetes, and cardiovascular diseases.

Flexible working time is the most effective strategy in dealing with the detrimental effects to people's social lives of modern work-life. In a study using over 21,000 European employees, it was shown that a high flexibility–low variability work schedule had positive affects, and confirmed growing evidence, that shift-work had a negative effect on sleep and the health of the employees. With proper alignment of your work and social times, you can look forward to improved health, well-being, and work satisfaction. What can you do now to help improve your situation?

Here is a list of job-related factors you need to be aware of and try to avoid:

- Shift-work (especially night-work)
- High workloads or overworking
- Over commitment to work
- Individual or team related problems
- A high perceived job stress level
- Job dissatisfaction
- Extra hours or duty days
- Irregular work schedules

Here are some tried and tested strategies and effective preventative measures, which will help you to improve your work-life balance:

- **A flexible work time** – this is principally earlier starts and later finishes in the summer months coupled with later starts and earlier finishes in the winter ones. It should also give you the opportunity to plan around important personal events and activities. The ability to govern your work load, perceived autonomy, and individualism in the workplace will leave you feeling positively motivated
- **Reduce working hours** – review your income and expenditure to see if by cutting a few extravagances out of your life you could not manage to reduce the numbers of hours you work
- **Real time management** – time management in the traditional sense should be avoided, as all it succeeds in doing is to accelerate the amount of work you do at the expense of the work quality, promotes an increase in personal pressures, and raises the expectations of you to artificially high and unsustainable levels. This activity should not be about listing as many things as you can to accomplish within an hour, day, week, or month. There is nothing more stressing than staring at a diary with appointments filled in every available slot from 8am to 8pm. A blank page maybe even worse, as it just screams out at you to fill it in with as many items as you can regardless of importance. It is not about to-do lists of valueless tasks either. Putting yourself under unnecessary pressure before you even start your day is the formula to stress and frustration, which will just reduce your work quality, work-life balance, and job satisfaction; an avoidable vicious circle.

14 Super steps to workplace productivity and peace!

1. Focus on tasks that allow a minimum of effort but return the highest rewards.
2. Planning your daily breaks is your first priority – reward yourself first.
3. Everything you do, from telephone calls to emails, from meetings to training, should have an identifiable purpose, measurable outcome, and a specific duration.
4. Any type of communication such as an email, letter, telephone call, voice mail, text message, or facsimile should be 'handled' just once. After the information is received you should:
    a. Action it immediately (minimum effort – maximum reward);
    b. File it or make of note of it;
    c. Forward it on to the relevant person/s;
    d. Trash it!
5. Aim for a clutter-free workstation; (easy on the eye is easy on the mind).
6. Your working capacity should be based around 60%. This allows time for thinking, planning, preparing, and reviewing.
7. In any project, you should always overestimate the time required to complete it, under-promise, and over-deliver the outcome.
8. Break larger projects into smaller chunks and seek to delegate the work, and utilise the skills and attributes of others to achieve more with less.
9. If available, always choose the easier options.
10. Leave difficult and disliked tasks until the middle of the day (sandwiched either side of tasks you enjoy or are proficient at completing).
11. Pass on your knowledge and experience at every available opportunity, and seek to mentor or coach people where possible.
12. Identify the 'helpers', 'positive influences', 'contrarians' and 'decision makers' and actively promote your interaction with them. Conversely, you should look to reduce your exposure to those people or things which are 'time-wasters', negative influences', and 'harbours of conflict'.
13. Avoid conflict and negative situations at all costs.
14. Be positive.

Chapter 14

Relax-tivity & MeTo opportunities

What kinds of thoughts do you conjure up when you hear or see the word 'relaxation'? It will mean different things to different people, but for most it will end up in some kind of mind-numbing, trance-like slouching (in front of the TV a usual favourite), a nap or sleeping, just doing nothing or as little as possible.

However, 'relaxing' should be viewed as an activity and one which is pursued and achieved, as oppose to something which is the result of eliminating as may actions or thoughts as you can. Relax-tivity is the marriage of 'relaxation' and 'activity'. The best sportspeople in the world, in their 'active' phases, will perform at their best when their muscles are 'relaxed', as a tension-filled muscle will produce an inferior performance. When you have the opportunity to watch good dancers, watch with marvel as they glide effortlessly across the ground, as if floating on air. This grace and guile is their ability to move without the hindrance of muscle and emotional tension. In contrast, a dancer lacking in such abilities will appear busy, hurried, jerky, and cumbersome; and incidentally not so pleasant viewing.

In the modern world people are constantly bombarded with an in surmountable level of information, informing them of the where, what, who, when, why, which, and how of just about everything. Most of the time, the filtered and processed information will only succeed in creating false hopes, unattainable dreams, and negative emotions, which all conspire to leave people with a longing for more; ultimately feeling unfulfilled and unhappy, and a proven road to poor health.

You need to have the ability to adapt to your personal circumstances and assist the repair and rejuvenation of your body. Sleep, as mentioned above and worth reiterating, is the undisputed master of repair and rejuvenation, and there is no substitute for it (not to be confused with sleep at any other time of day). Relax-tivity, however, if used in conjunction with the appropriate amount of good quality sleep, will encompass mind and body benefiting activities such as breathing and meditative activities, physical activity, positive thinking, radiant people, visualisation, self-massage, music, smell, and the natural environment to establish 'my essential time-out' (MeTo) opportunities. MeTo will be easily accessible and will provide the tools to your continued health and well-being.

There are four basic underlying components of Relax-tivity, which when combined create the foundation for peace of mind and good health:

- **Attentiveness**
- **Simplicity**
- **Sensitivity**
- **Balancing**

Attentiveness – Be aware of the stresses and strains, which act on your mind and body; look out for wellness inhibitors such as poor body alignment and posture, inefficient breathing practices, incorrect body movements and the more obvious signs such as illness, aches, or pains. Paying attention to the smallest details will ensure that any warning signs emitted will be picked up and larger problems will be foreseen and acted on.

In addition, you have a very powerful intuitive sense; this sense is unexpected, and can occur in a sudden and immediate fashion, with no seemingly logical explanation. The word 'intuition' comes from the Latin *intueri*, meaning to look within; this powerful internal tool is the ability to 'read' the situation, with ingredients consisting of information received from the five body senses and a illogical sprinkling of faith! Being receptive to this valuable knowledge and insight facilitates your attentiveness and empowers you to be proactive in your quest for good health and wellness.

Simplicity – Use minimum effort to create maximum health. Maximum health or vitality is achieved by not wasting valuable mental or physical energy. Every word, thought, or action requires energy, so it is paramount to ensure everything you do is both functional and purposeful. Using the 80/20 principle as outlined in Richard Koch's book, Living the 80/20 Way, you can achieve 80% of what you want in life with only 20% of the effort – so why waste the remaining 80% of effort trying to seek the 100%?. This is a truly magical principle and by attaching it to the way, you live create an environment of powerful simplicity. The author's message can be summed up in three words: More with Less. Think of how effortlessly a champion canoeist will negotiate the most volatile of rivers with the minimum of effort; tuning themselves into the forces and contours of the waves in order to experience greater fluidity of motion, as if a part of the river itself. However, simplicity is not just passively going with the flow, as the canoeist, is in control of the situation (the choice of route, effort exerted, etc.). Seek this kind of simplicity to live with a laser-like focus and concentration, two powerful attributes to increase your vitality and maximise your energy with a minimum of effort.

Sensitivity – Is your ability to detect the slight changes in yourself, the people around you, and your immediate environment. This will allow you to observe changes and their reactions as they occur, empowering you to address situations as they arise, and return to some kind of emotional and/or physical balance before they spiral out of control, or are unnecessarily prolonged. It is good practice to live with the principle that feelings and emotions are better dealt with out in the open, as oppose to, suppressed within. Any kind of suppression will magnify the power of that feeling, which will eventually manifest itself in a more potent way, such as, an illness or disease, or in the shape of negative emotions such as, anger and anxiety. Family, friends, and partners in everyday situations provide the perfect examples of where a little more sensitivity would supply a more peaceful and content environment to live in. Think of the times, when you are confronted by a person who just seems to 'snap' into a rage or let fly a few negative and critical remarks for no apparent reason. The signs preceding this kind of event are always available and it is in a person's power to avert such situations before they arise, if they practice sensitivity.

Two important activities need to be practiced regularly in order to establish good sensitivity: observation and listening. For instance, observing body language provides the visual flags, and listening to what and the way things are said, provides the auditory ones, which when added together will help decipher the emotional and physical status of yourself and others in time to avert prolonging a detrimental situation. You should aim to, if not already, for your future peace and happiness, master the mannerisms of your family, friends, and partner.

Balancing – As with everything in your body and environment, it is a question of maintaining balance. Your vitality can be positively correlated with the ability and speed with which you return to balance from the emotional swings (be they positive, such as euphoria and excitement sensations or negative ones, such as stress, anger, and frustration) and the physical strains and tensions of everyday life. Maintaining balance is about your perception and belief, and how you choose to react to the situations you encounter in life. You may choose to inflate, raise the importance, create a nightmare scenario, be negative, or complicate the situation. Alternatively, you could choose the road to vitality and inner peace by reducing the impact, depth, and duration of any emotional and physical swings. Balancing allows you to view or perceive a situation from the many different angles always available, which then give you the opportunity to re-balance the situation into context. To practice balancing when faced with difficult situations, you need to:

- be positive in your thinking
- dispel overblown and nightmare scenarios; as 90% of what you think is going to happen never actually does
- rank the situation and reduce its importance; play it down as it will very rarely be that important
- simplify the situation into smaller parts; the situation will seem less daunting and easier to deal with
- consult and request the help of others; there will always be someone somewhere who has successfully gone through similar situations or knows of someone who has
- identify solutions; a solution goal will move you closer to the solution you want
- be flexible; as there are also more than one solution to any given situation

Actively seeking a return to body and emotional balance is rewarded exponentially with vitality and well-being; it will deter any manifestations of prolonged exaggeration and negativity, or any reductions in your energy, which only combine to increase your chances of illness and disease.

How do you use Relax-tivity?
You can always do with some time to yourselves, your very own 'personal care islands', where you can take mental and physical repair and rejuvenation holidays. Easy access to these kinds of holidays is rare, so you have to create them for yourself. This is the opportunity to say "MeTo!" and take one of those holidays to those increasingly elusive personal care islands. You can use the components of Relax-tivity: attentiveness, sensitivity, simplicity, and balancing, to introduce into your everyday life, highly potent stress busting and mood elevating MeTo opportunities, and gain daily fixes of, not only, peace and tranquillity but also inner-strength and vitality.

Here are the top ten most effective MeTo opportunities to transport you to your personal care islands:

The Ultimate Ten - MeTo opportunities

1. Breathing activities: Breathing is the most important function of your life, and you should take the appropriate amount of time to perfect it. Breathing activities can be performed anywhere and at anytime to give you the power to live with increased energy, vitality, and mental focus; reduced stress levels; strengthened immune system; renewed body parts and invigorated body functions; and reversed premature aging. (Refer to Part one – Breath of life).

2. Meditative activities: Breathing activities can be meditative, as can physical activity. In fact, there is no limit to the number of situations which you cannot attach some kind of meditative benefit. There needs to be a move away from the idea that meditation is only about empting the mind of all thoughts, or one that can only be performed in perfect silence and tranquil surroundings. It should not be viewed as a mystical or magical art form, which takes years of training to perform or one that is only practiced by a few elite peoples around the world, or one that has many rules that need to be adhered to. You have the capability to perform meditative activities and what is more, can perform them in your everyday lives while doing everyday activities, and reap the benefits involved. Meditative activities can be incorporated into life such as when walking, gardening, doing domestic tasks, eating, standing in a queue, observing nature, listening to music, dancing, or playing an instrument.

Lu Lin, working mother of three, would always complain of not having the time or patience for things like meditation. Citing the fact that any spare time was spent with, or clearing up after, her children (aged two, three, and five). Lu Lin was introduced to the concept of daily meditative activities she could incorporate into her existing routines. Her daily journey to work was the starting point. On leaving the house I asked her to, while maintaining a constant and deliberate breathing pattern and rate, concentrate and focus on the methodical and rhythmic walking action; breaking the action down into its smallest parts; the heel hitting the ground followed by the sole of the foot, and the toes; alternating focus between left foot and right. At the station while waiting for the train (whether seated or standing) she concentrated on her breathing rate and pattern, and shifted her weight from one foot to the other (unnoticeable to others at the station) in time with her breathing. While on the train, I would ask her to, where possible, close her eyes and paint vivid mental images of places of natural beauty she had visited (or would like to visit). If closing her eyes were not an option, then I would ask her to choose a point of focus inside the train, (as pointlessly staring out of the window would only cram useless mental images and references into her subconscious mind), and continue to practice good breathing. The techniques used are very simple, and the simplicity of such adaptable and effective techniques continues to help Lu Lin to MeTo opportunities everyday.

3. Physical activity: Activities such as walking, dancing, gardening, and vigorous housework, as well as having meditative aspects, all carry supreme health and well being benefits. If you were to perform these types of activities on a daily basis, you can expect benefits such as an increased control over your weight, a strengthened internal and external body (such as improved heart, lung function, stronger muscles and bones), greater flexibility, an enhanced immune system, and an improved standard of health. This in itself is a very important and integral part of your existence and is therefore the subject of Part five – Made for motion.

4. Positive thinking: You are 100% responsible for all the emotions you experience and it is the way you 'choose' to see things, which create the pathway to your future.

> I don't get depressed; I grow a tumour instead.
>
> *Woody Allen*

When you are positive in thought, everything in life has the capacity to work well. Your choice to view a situation in either a positive or a negative way (as there are very few instances where a person does not feel either one or other) probably costs you the same amount of energy for either thought process. However, the aftermath of such thoughts create either an uplifting mood or a downward spiralling one to suffering. You have both positive and negative pre-programmed reactions to certain situations, which occur on autopilot, which are picked up from your experiences in childhood, from parents, and from the relationships with others, amongst other things. How do you change the negative automatic reactions?

Firstly, the good news is that you can change them. Secondly, the steps to change are relatively straightforward and simple to follow. Identify the situations and events of where you usually choose to be negative. This preparation will provide you with the awareness you need to be proactive and forearmed with positive thoughts and actions. In addition, if you use visualisation (refer to MeTo opportunity number six) you can 'relive' negative beliefs and your pre-programmed reactions as though they are recordings on a camcorder, making it easier to change them and record new positive ones in their place; the key is to view each situation with 'new eyes' as they arise.

How do you change the negative automatic reactions?

- Acknowledge the negative thoughts as your own (without trying to be self-critical or trying to blame others)
- Defuse the situation by using the question "How could the situation be worse?" By getting as many negative scenarios out of your system as you can, will actually take you closer to a positive one
- Offer positive facts
- Reward yourself for your successful actions; be good to yourself

Here is how a friend described the way he managed his moment of negativity using this system:

> I was driving to a job interview for a senior banking position at one of the world top-five investment banks and had given myself plenty of time for the journey. The traffic started to slow down, and before I knew it, I was surrounded by stationary cars. Cars moved a metre every five minutes or so. I knew this because my eyes would repeatedly scan the clock in the car and the watch on my wrist (just in case there was an error between the two). Even though it was a cold winter's day, the first signs of sweat appeared on my forehead after about fifteen minutes. On looking in the rear-view mirror, I noticed my face features starting to contort and I was noticeably red. I was gripping the steering wheel tighter and tighter as time passed. My neck disappeared as my shoulders tightened towards my ears. I was berating myself with barrage after barrage of criticism and could think of nothing else other than how very important an interview this was for me and I just had to get there on time.
>
> This had to stop. I made the decision to change and used your positive thinking formula to do it. Firstly, I acknowledged all the negative thoughts and the self-criticism such as where did all these people come from, I should have left earlier, planned a better route, recharged by mobile phone last night, chosen another time for the interview, should not have applied for the job in the first place, and I don't deserve the job anyway. This activity in itself was starting to release some of my tensions, as it made me realise how much I was beating-up on myself. 'How could it be worse?' Well, this was when my imagination went into overdrive and I rattled off multiple worse-situation scenarios: it could have been snowing; I could be trapped for days; my car could be filled with crying children; the radio could

be stuck on a heavy metal station; my ex-wife could be in the car. This went on for another few minutes or so (because I was not actually tracking the time anymore). The next two steps were the icing on the cake and after completing them, I was uplifted and much happier. 'Offer positive facts' allowed me to list all the things that were great in my life at that time such as the fact I was in a new loving relationship, had just made up with my brother, was in good health, and was in fact good enough to even be considered for this fantastic role. Finally, I needed to reward myself for 'choosing' to be positive; I promised myself a three-day break in the countryside.

My friend was late by four hours and was not interviewed for the job. He nevertheless chose to give his explanation as to why he was so late in person, and even though the Partner and Manager were 'unavailable', he proceeded to give it to one of their personal assistants, who was sympathetic but also at a loss as to why he was so happy about it! A few months later, he had secured another interview and is currently working for a rival investment bank in the building next door (and is now an ardent user of public transport).

Positive thinking is a step towards a happier and healthier outlook on life, whereas negative thoughts will take you closer to stress, illness, and disease. Life is full of challenges, so why choose to perceive the situations you will face with negativity. You need to be honest with yourself and acknowledge the fact that most of your negative thoughts regarding a given situation will never actually happen, so why worry about them in the first place and use up valuable supplies of good health.

5. Radiant people: It is highly likely that you have met and enjoyed the benefits of many radiant people in your life, whether aware of it or not. As a successful international Wellness Consultant, I had the opportunities to travel often and my appointments ranged from executive consultations and corporate presentations to group FAT (Functional Activity Training) sessions, and sports team conditioning programs. These opportunities afforded me many meetings with radiant people. It is important to note that they are just ordinary people and the kind you are likely to bump into at any point in your life. They seem to emit an uplifting energy that is like the warm glow of an open fireplace, and communicating with or just being in the presence of these people will always leave you in a refreshed and reenergised state. You can spot these people because they always seem to be in a positive mood, smiling, cheerful, and seemingly without a care in the world and thankfully, neither their education level or financial status has any bearing on their positive radiance.

Here are a few simple steps to help you increase your MeTo opportunities with radiant people:

- Identify those (by using the Relax-tivity component: Sensitivity) who emit this positive renewing energy
- Share and nurture connections with as many people as you can who emit this positive renewing energy (as the more people you can connect with the greater your levels of health and happiness)
- Increase (within reason) the frequency and duration of time you spend with them
- Avoid situations of take, take, take, otherwise negativity will eventually manifest itself, negating any positive effects of your connections
- You can use all forms of communication to nurture and cultivate these connections
- Most children are great sources of positive renewing energy (and entertaining ones too!)

Conversely, you will feel a negative radiance when, for example, if your partner has had a rotten day, you have had an intense argument, or in the presence of an 'energy sponge'. An encounter with an energy sponge is not about good vibes and positive energy. It is in fact, a reversal of energy flow, and I have had my fair share of encounters with them. You can experience this reversal of energy flow with people (who I would like to think are completely unaware of the effect they have), animals or places.

> The greater part of the fatigue from which we suffer is of mental origin.
>
> *J.A. Hadfield*
> *The psychology of power*

Let me share a typical experience that occurred when I was consulting in Istanbul. The client was a major finance company executive and after an initial consultation, it was agreed that weekly sessions (two to three a week) would bring them closer to there goals in the fastest and safest way. Below is a brief history of the client (the personal details have been altered to protect privacy):

> Hale Yilmaz lived in rented accommodation in the affluent area of Istanbul. Her commute to work was forty minutes each way on an overcrowded public bus. Her day normally started at 6am

with a hurried cup of coffee with little or no breakfast. On autopilot, she would reach her desk by 7.30am, having grabbed another coffee and a quick bite of anything that looked appealing along the way. A lunch, snack, litres of water, another snack, a few cups of coffee, and a basket of stresses and crises later, it would be time to go home. These were the daily highlights and there was not much for Hale to be enthusiastic about her work. She declared that she disliked her role within the finance company and had been actively seeking new employment for eighteen months, nonetheless would normally arrive at home at around 8pm.

She would regularly complained of headaches, body pains, lethargy, fatigue, constant minor ailments, and depressive mood swings, as was her inability to maintain her perceived ideal weight. She had great difficulty in sleeping on most nights and took medication to help her sleep. She admits that socially she has very few 'real' friends and does not have ideal relationships with her family. She will rarely speak to anybody else after she has left work. In her personal relationships, she complains it is hard to meet people and even harder to maintain a loving one, pointing at the string of broken friendships for no apparent reasons, as evidence. At thirty-two she felt the 'next one' has to be 'the' one, as she felt she was under body time constraints, parental and peer pressure, and unable to leave things to chance.

At first, I was unaware of the effect these sessions would have on me, and would just put it down to general tiredness because the sessions always took place in the evening. As time passed, I began to observe a pattern in my energy levels and matched the energy declines to these sessions. Hale's attitude to most things was negative and defeatist, with little room for optimism or joy. Conversely, my attitude is positive and hopeful and actively tries to extract simple pleasures from a complex life. Even though I would always actively listen to her, be observant without being judgemental and supportive without being patronising, my heart rate would rise and my breathing patterns would be short and shallow. A tension would fill my muscles and I exhibited visuals clues of frustration such as pen tapping, fidgeting, and awkward cumbersome movements. As I gave, she took; the more I gave, the more she took. As my emotional and physical energy was being siphoned away, I would feel drained and exhausted.

Here is how to reduce your time with energy sponges:

- Identify those who leave you mentally exhausted and with reduced energy levels
- Break or cease connections with as many of these people as you can
- Decrease the frequency and duration of time you spend with them if you are unable to completely break-free
- Avoid situations of give, give, give; it is unhealthy

6. Visualisation: This is the ability to produce mental images, which sharpen awareness, and sensitivity, and empowers a change in the way a person mentally or physically reacts to events and situations. It should not be confused with night or daydreams and visions, which are usually symbolic and complicated manifestations of something that has been experienced or being experienced (which can be useful for something completely different). Visualisation is a type of training in focus and concentration, which has been practised for hundreds of years. It uses the creative power of the mind, to substitute positive images for negative ones, as a healing power for illness and disease (practised in both the East and the West). It helps to help cure addictions and phobias, reduce stress levels, as pre-emptive preparation for any situation (such as an interview, examination, speech, difficult conversation, sporting events, or diplomacy and negotiations), and to increase both emotional and physical strength and resolve.

Every action of your body is the result of some kind of internal chemistry; the brain is affected by neurotransmitters such as serotonin and dopamine, while the body functions are regulated by hormones, like adrenaline and testosterone. The activity in your brain controls the release of hormones by the glands into your blood, which regulates body functions such as energy production, metabolism, and are involved in the control of emotional, sexual, and your other behaviours. Hormones carried up to the brain in your blood will then serve to influence the activity of the brain itself.

This is the key to the power of visualisation; as the brain is unaware of the differences between something you experience in real-life compared to something that is vividly imagined, and will therefore send out emotional or physical messages as if you had actually experienced the event or situation. Think of something you are afraid of, such as a snake, spider, or dog. If you were to imagine a time, where you are confronted by one of these creatures in true cinematic colour, sound and visuals, your brain, and body would react as if it were real. You would 'feel' fearful, and start to display body reactions to that fear such as an increased heart rate, knotting in the stomach, and perspiration, even though you were not actually experiencing it. How do you use visualisation?

Here are five steps to help you use the creative power of your mind to achieve what you desire:

1. Decide what you want and write it down in as much detail as you can; having a specific and predefined goal or solution will help you achieve it
2. Use your imagination to 'smell, taste, touch, see and feel' yourself achieving the goal or solution you want; your images should be as vivid, colourful, emotional, and engaging as possible to extract 'real' responses from your mental and physical functions
3. Rehearse it over and over again
4. Make it real!
5. Review the progress to your desired goal or solution; make any minor adjustments as necessary. Go to step 2

Meet Maria an experienced professional volleyball player based in Barcelona, Spain; and one of her goals was to improve her game. She was in very good shape and her physical preparation was, as what you would expect of a professional athlete. Her game however would seem to falter towards the end of sets (the business end of the game if you asked her coach), and this was having an adverse effect on her confidence, which was then reducing the standard of her game; a vicious circle. At her first consulting session with me, Maria wrote down in good detail exactly the way she wanted to perform. Taking this goal, I got Maria to imagine as if she were watching herself on a big TV screen; she could see herself making diving plays, perfect spikes, and winning serves; she could see and hear the crowd and her coach, enjoy the hugs of her congratulating teammates. She was actually 'living' the way she wanted. Maria went away after a few more sessions and practised her visualisation before each match.

What was the outcome to her training? Throughout the year, telephone sessions helped Maria to fine-tune her visualisations and allow her to provide feedback of her feelings and performances. She reported that confidence levels had increased and was making fewer errors in matches (compared to the season before). At the end of the season, Maria was given her first Most Improved Player award. Moreover, it did not stop there as she started to use the visualisation techniques in other parts of her life, such as her salary and contract negotiations, and personal relationships.

7. Self-massage: The chronic overload and overuse of muscles in a person's daily life is commonplace, for example, at work, a person will tend to assume poor body positions, postures, and perform repetitive tasks, all of which create avoidable muscle strains and tensions. Other factors, which can put an unnecessary stress on your muscles and cause pain, include being overweight, not partaking in regular and varied physical activity, and suffering from forms of stress, tension, or anxiety. Stretching exercises, hot and cold remedies, or such like, may produce a temporary relief from the pain for a tightened or tense muscle, but they will rarely produce a positive long-term solution. The safest and most effective method to treat the aches and pains accumulated in your body is deep stroke massage. This type of massage is perfectly adaptable to self-massage and promotes a stronger immune system, improved circulation, reduces the risks of injury, makes you move and feel better, and revitalizes your energy levels.

Why self-massage? There is no need to wait for an appointment, treat your ailments whenever you want in your own comfortable surroundings, it does not cost any money (making it accessible to everyone), and removes the guess work required in trying to tell someone what is causing the pain, or where it is. Who is in the best possible position to know how you feel? You are! You are the expert of your own body (or should learn to be) and be in direct control over your treatment. Self-massage should be an integral part of your personal wellness plan; it can cure a wide ranging list of aches and pains such as earaches, headaches, muscular pains (neck, arms, back, legs, shoulders, etc.), dizziness, nausea, sleeplessness, fatigue, and heartburn. Incidentally, you should always seek a non-drug remedy wherever possible for any such ailments and reduce the need of painkillers for the relief of pain.

Your self-massage guidelines:

- Use a massage tool where you can (especially for shoulder, back, lower back, and buttocks)
- Use deep stroke massage; work your fingers deep, slow, and with very short strokes. Think of your muscle as though it were dough and you need to knead your way along it
- Work in one direction only
- All strokes towards the heart. The direction of your kneading massage action should move you towards the heart. For instance, working your calf, leg, and arm muscles will mean your strokes move upward; or for neck muscles, the strokes will be downward.

- Be systematic in your approach. Your muscle is like a stringed harp, you need to touch each string to effect the treatment
- Massage the areas close to the ache or pain you are suffering. Most of the time, an ache or pain is the end points of a tension or strain somewhere close by, for example, a headache can be caused by a pain in the neck muscles.*
- Perform your self-massage daily

*For a comprehensive listing of body pains, and where they originate from, refer to the extensive in-depth reference books available in most libraries Myofascial Pain and Dysfunction: The Trigger Point Manuals Vol. 1 & 2 by Travell & Simons.

8. Music: It has the power to make you toe-tap, head-nod, and deliriously dance; it can calm, soothe, and relax you; evoke sadness, irritation, and anger; transport you to a time in your past and heal you in the future. A great return on the investment of the price of a CD!

Music is a very powerful tool you can use to affect your physical and mental well-being; it can reduce stress-like symptoms, provide inner strength and peace, and evoke strong reactions. However, it is also very personal and very difficult to prescribe from person to person. For example, your average teenager may be listening to what's 'hot' in the music charts, extracting good feelings and be thoroughly entertained by it, while an older person may be irritated by it. Moreover, it is not just cross-age bands either, as people of the same age and similar backgrounds may take the complete opposite views of a music gender; one loves jazz and is exhilarated and energised by it, while the other hates it and is depressed by it.

Various clients used music to reach their desired state; Richard a marathon runner would choose composers like Handel, Beethoven, and Bach, to calm and focus for competitive races. Whereas Michael, a seasoned American Football player preferred to listen to rap music for its aggressive attitude and no-nonsense approach. Margaret, a police officer in a very busy Los Angeles neighbourhood could be found dancing out of her uniform and into her civil clothes to the beat of a random 80's disco / funk song.

The key is to know what kind of music puts you into what mood and then use it accordingly. Making compilations of different songs from different albums is now very easy due to advancing technology and the way you can purchase and record music. To get the maximum impact from music, create compilations for specific purposes. For instance, if you are soothed and calmed by listening to classical music then bring together a collection of your favourite compositions to one source, and use it in times of stress and tension. Or if your brother is coming to visit and bringing the five children along (for his entertainment), then the 'never-say-die' attitude of about twenty back-to-back rock tracks may be just what you need to motivate and energise you before they arrive.

Music used in this way are perfect MeTo opportunities, but please use the power wisely and considerately, as your music may be noise pollution (and consequently unhealthy) to others.

9. Smell: Sense of smell, in the earlier days for humans, was used to detect foods, individuals (be they friend, foe, or the opposite sex), territory, as well as dangers. A person has the capacity to smell many different odours but only one odour at a time, as stronger odours will overpower weaker ones. This sense of smell can evoke emotional and physical reactions, which result in strong approach or avoidance behaviours. The smell of freshly cut grass or baked bread will bring pleasure as oppose to that of smelly feet or rotting trash, causing nausea.

Today, there is increased access to aromatherapy treatments, which can promote health and well-being; it uses the power of smell to heal, calm, relieve, rejuvenate, heighten sensitivity, and uplift moods. Use the following pleasing and natural oil fragrances to put you in your desired state:

- Calm and soothing: lavender; rose; cypress, chamomile
- De-stress and pacifying: lemon balm; sage; orange
- Energising: lemon; eucalyptus; cinnamon
- Alert and focused: clove; peppermint; rosemary
- Uplifting: jasmine; fennel; basil

As a bonus, you can also use good quality oils such as almond, for skin care, room scenting, massage, and perfume. The wide ranging sources and differing scented oils are perfect replacements for the oversold, overused, and extortionately overpriced chemically laced equivalents you will find in the shops today; you would need to be a bona fide chemist to recall or understand the ingredients of most skin care creams, lotions, or potions.

10. The natural environment: In actively seeking to improve your health and well-being, it is important to take special note of how the environment affects you and what you can do about it. Let me first share some of the feelings I experience on the very special occasions I get the opportunity to visit friends and family in Cyprus. The small Mediterranean island of love and beauty is a stepping-stone between the Middle East and Europe, and it is my emotional and physical haven, where I can find balance. The abundance of space, nature, natural beauty, white sands, and sky blue seas positively feed my depleted emotional and physical energy supplies. I will usually walk on the nearby beach or through the abundance supply of olive groves and always take the time to devour the smallest detail while sucking on the fresh air and absorbing the scenery. After a successful walk, any negative energy would be released from by body, as if it were as easy as turning on a tap and watching the stresses flow out of my feet. All of my senses are engaged, and yet I would feel calm, revitalised, and replenished with positive energy.

Surprisingly for some, I would also engage similar emotions and benefits when I was in an expansive metropolis, such as London. Finding the time to rebalance in a non-stop city can prove difficult, but I would always find time in between appointments to visit anyone of the great public parks and open spaces there. When in Central London, my favourite place was Regents Park, which cast a large green five-kilometre circumference net in the middle of the concrete jungle. It was lavished with beautifully manicured gardens, open green spaces, and a large pond at one end with a London Zoo at the other, which meant you could always find a spot to revitalise. The place for me was the bench close to the bandstand (not in use at the time) overlooking the pond where the ducks and swans would take up most of my attention as I observed their individual mannerisms.

Interacting with your natural environment is an amazingly simple, yet thoroughly effective way to increase your own peace, tranquillity, inner strength, and vitality. For those lucky enough to live in natural surroundings know exactly what I am referring to. For those who live in urban surroundings, you should seek the solace of places such as parks, gardens, and tranquil areas to extract their natural vitality (as well as trying to sneak out of town to enjoy Mother Nature at every available opportunity). To make the most of your MeTo opportunities and not let them pass by without savouring them or without achieving your own 'natural high', you should ensure that you:

- spend some time in nature; a park, garden, fields, beach, seaside, mountains, rooftop garden, tranquil areas, etc
- observe the surroundings and try to concentrate on a few simple things with an eye on the detail
- use changes in weather and seasons to create new experiences

Part five

Made for motion

Physical activity is something you are born to do, it is part of your genetic make-up, and the mechanics of which have evolved over millions of years; just as fish swim, birds fly, you are at your most efficient when performing an activity such as walking. Modern life has provided an abundance of food to eat, increased calorie consumptions, and deprived people of ways and reasons to be physically active, decreasing energy expenditure.

This imbalance in your energy formula has opened the door on a host of modern illnesses, diseases, and increased rates of mortality. Physical inactivity reduces your quality of life preventing you from living the way you would like to. It is a conscious choice toward a slow suicide. Being physically active is, without doubt, of great importance in the quest for health, well-being, quality of life, and longevity. Physical activity coupled with nourishment represent the formula for body energy, as the former accounts for energy expenditure, and the later, energy intake. In Part three - Nourishment, the importance of what is eaten, and how big an impact it has on health and well-being has already been identified and proved.

When the words 'physical activity' are used throughout this book, and especially in the following chapters, it is referring to any body movement produced by muscle action which increases energy expenditure; activities such as walking, gardening, climbing stairs, hiking, carrying groceries, light manual DIY, leisure activities, and housework. It does not refer to 'exercise' a subset of physical activity which is planned, structured, repetitive body conditioning movements which are repeated over time (days, weeks, durations, and intensities) such as most activities at fitness centres or gyms (treadmill, stair master, cross-trainer, stationary bike, rowing machines, resistance machines, aerobics classes, etc.). These types of exercises only serve to restrict your body movements and do not allow for natural free-flowing ranges of movement. This constrictive and repeating nature of exercise can be violent and damaging on the body parts; and by adding long durations and high intensities to this type of exercise, it only succeeds in promoting unnecessary exhaustion or unnatural fatigue. This can be viewed as more of an injury as oppose to an advantage, as the overworked body parts just create an excessive waste of energy (instead of increasing it). By being inactive for most of the day or week, you will be doing yourself harm and a disservice if you think you can make-up for the physical activity deficiencies (or excessive food and drink consumption) in sessions of excessive exercise (despite what the multi-billion profit-making fitness industry would like you to believe).

The following pages will cover the body's need for physical activity and how it promotes the optimal performance of all your body systems (such as the muscles, bones, heart, lungs, neural, digestive, hormonal, immune, and blood), to improve well-being, reduce stress, and increase your years of purposeful living.

Chapter 15

Body basics

Evolving over the past million or so years, humans have been genetically programmed for mobility; the overall genetic makeup of Homo sapiens has changed little during the past 10,000 years, and are still genetically adapted to a pre-agricultural hunter-gatherer life-style. Hunter-gatherer societies would have required a fundamental need for moderate physical activity in order to provide the necessities of life, such as food, water, shelter, materials for warmth, in order to survive.

Consequently, the human body is an efficient two-legged locomotive structure. The upright posture also afforded the Homo sapiens other benefits such as freeing their hands for tools and weapons, and a higher vantage point with which to spot food or danger. When walking your two-legged motion uses a toggle-like action making the energy transfer more efficient than in the legs of four-legged mammals. The skeletal frame, shape, and dimension together with the muscles form the largest part of your total body mass. A body will utilise skeletal muscles to move; and there are about 700 of them in varying shapes, sizes, and strengths. Muscles are supported in their ability to provide your locomotion by the diverse structural and mechanical functions of the skeleton, and its various joints and levers. The skeleton comprises of 206 bones in various sizes, weight, and shapes which provides many variations of movement, as well as functions such as protection, support, and storage. Although you have a very versatile and resilient structure, the power and efficiency is in your legs, the muscles found here are the strongest and longest ones. Not only do they allow you to move with great economy but are also the pillars of your stability and posture.

You are built to use walking as a mode of transport (previously used to fulfil the hunter-gatherer way of life). When humans (or primates) run, it is usually due to the adoption of the 'fight or flight' instincts in order to escape confrontation or danger; however, this emergency mode of transport is inefficient in comparison to walking. When humans (or primates) run, it costs almost twice as much energy as it does for four-legged mammals.

Nearly 100% of human existence has been dominated by outdoor physical activity, but unlike some other animals who when introduced into this world have the ability to walk and run (especially in the event of danger), human independence and mobility takes a little more time to mature. When born, humans are helpless and have no other alternative than to stay very close to the nurturing hands of parents. Only after a couple of years of nurturing can humans stand on their own two-feet!

> Our children are spontaneously physically active (if we
> allowed them to be) and so were we…once upon a time.
> *Health-Warrior*

In the fall of 2002, I visited one of the few peoples and places left on this Earth, while travelling between Botswana and Namibia, where people still follow the hunter-gatherer lifestyle; the Bushmen of the Kalahari Desert. It was a chance to observe a way of life thousands of years old, and gave me the opportunity to contrast the differences with the modern way of living. Their days were filled with trying to gather a sufficient amount of food, which meant fast walking for long distances when hunting, or digging, and squatting like actions when foraging for berries, roots, and various other plants. Before nightfall, it was a question of finding firewood for cooking, light, and warmth. The Bushmen are physically active, and it is not of their want to be healthy or to be in better physical shape, but their drive is initiated by their need for food and water.

In an article 'Every Day is a Gift When You Are 100' published by the National Geographic Society a few decades ago, scientist Alexander Leaf visited the regions of the world where some people were said to regularly live past a hundred years, and remained relatively untouched by the modern world. All the regions were remote and mountainous: the Andean village of Vilcabamba in Ecuador, the land of Hunza in the Karakoram Range in Pakistani-controlled Kashmir, and Abkhazia in the old Georgian Soviet Socialist Republic in the southern Soviet Union.

> I was amazed at such exertion by a man over a hundred, but
> wherever I went, the level of physical activity among such old
> people was high.
> *Alexander Leaf, M.D.*

Indeed, many lived well into old age, and had its fair share of centenarians. These older people of all three cultures displayed remarkable levels of physical activity, with both men and women employed in the vigour of traditional farming and household chores from early childhood to their terminal days. They also walked a great deal and considering their mountainous habitat, was a feat in itself that promoted high degrees of cardiovascular fitness as well as general muscular tone.

At around the same time, David Davies and his team, also had the good fortune to explore the relatively remote and mountainous area of Vilcabamba and the surrounding areas of southern Ecuador. In his subsequent book, 'The Centenarians of the Andes' published in 1975, he detailed how the Ecuadorians lived much longer and were more physically active in old age than when compared to the modern societies of back then. He went on to highlight the significances of life in the highlands of the Andes, and reports that its people live longer; are free of killer diseases such as cancer, heart disease, and diabetes; and are physically active and in command of all their faculties. The Ecuadorians, Davies observed, walk a great deal in and around their mountainous villages; and it was this activity, which he concluded, was the foundation of their excellent health and well-being.

> If one does not use a machine, it becomes rusty. If one sits in a chair the whole time, at what is considered to be the end of one's days, the parts are bound to seize up, simply through lack of use. Keeping working and active helps the vital body fluids to circulate, and keeps the muscles toned up and in good condition. The blood supply will then be driven to all parts of the body and, in doing so, it feeds and renews the body cells... 'Without rest, a man cannot work; without work, the rest does not give you benefit.' [An Ecuadorian saying]
>
> *David Davies*
> *The Centenarians of the Andes*

Ancient activity
Various cultures at differing periods in human existence have all shown concern for physical activity and the benefits they associated with it. The evolution of physical activity has been well documented in history and the practices and the beliefs of which can still be observed today.

In ancient China, its people were drawn to the disciplines such as T'ai chi, for conditioning of the mind and body and martial art disciplines, such as Kung fu or Wu Gong, for its personal protection. Personal protection was used in its widest sense of meaning, the ability to defend oneself from human or animal attack, protect oneself from illness and disease, and to find inner peace and well-being. Over the few thousand years that the Chinese have been practising the martial art activities, it was observed that individuals who were physically active on a regular basis were healthier than those who were inactive. The Wu Gong martial art is an example of the thousands of active styles of Qigong. Qigong can be translated as 'working with the energy of life', which is an integrated mind-body healing method displaying remarkable results in its effectiveness to heal and prevent illness and disease. The actions and techniques of those who practised Wu Gong resulted in better health and improved performance long into old age. The dynamic martial art improved the functions of the body, such as strength and flexibility in those who practised it. In modern-day China, this form of martial art is still practised and is still one of the most popular activities in promoting good health and well-being.

At around similar times, people of ancient India would practise variations of yoga. Matters of the mind carried high levels of importance for the Hindu and Buddhist alike. Yoga was seen as physical activity, which married the mind and body and secured the internal and external benefits for a healthier existence. Yoga has many differing styles and practises but is generally a series of postures and activities that incorporate regulated breathing, concentration, strength, and flexibility. The health benefits of yoga continue to be experienced today and most styles are no different from those practised thousands of years ago.

Pitting the strength of one man against another was the motivational force behind the physical activities of the ancient Egyptians and Persians. Preparing an army for battle meant special emphasis on the health of its soldiers; physical activities promoting strength and endurance (and incorporating the use of weapons) were regularly practised. Males were trained in the techniques of war from a very early age and often at the expense of any schooling, as it was deemed that a soldier did not require to be educated in order to protect his country. The link between the body and mind not holding a high level of importance in this era, so it was more a question of 'brawn' over 'brain'.

The ancient Greeks reintroduced the view that physical activity was just as important as education. An ancient Greek could be found reading books, as well as, practising activities, which promoted their improved physical health. Physical activity was very important for the Greeks, and as a result they introduced the worlds first Olympic Games. The Games by virtue of the fact that the contestants appeared nude meant that the contest itself became more a work of art; where artists and sculptors drew inspiration from it, (the evidence of such inspiration is freely available in the museums of today). This was a true spectator event, where the external beauty of the human structure grew to be more important than its prowess or its strength, and physical activity became training in aesthetics as much as, or more than, in physical excellence.

Unlike the ancient Greeks, ancient Romans had a double-edged view of the value of a physically fit person; of course, the health benefits it offered to the individual but also because of the benefits it provided for the empire. Physically mentally fit and healthier people made better soldiers and workers, and helped the government protect and expand the empire. Ancient Romans preferred to witness the glory of a victor who had competed in professional games and were not very interested if there was not a material reward on offer.

So even this very brief look back at the peoples of ancient times provides clues and helpful hints in the search for better health; to this extent, it can be said that better health (physical or mental) is elevated to a higher level if physical activity is a fundamental component of it.

Chapter 16

Curse of inactivity

Modern living has spawned a society where people seem to seesaw between the permanent excess of over-working, over-eating, and over-spending, and a sedentary one. This swinging between excess and scarcity is having a destructive impact on health and well-being. Industrialised societies have, knowingly or unknowingly, systematically excluded physical activity from daily lives. Even walking the simplest and most natural of all activities can require the skills and protective wear of a slalom skier.

> We sit at breakfast, we sit on the train on the way to work, we sit at work, we sit at lunch, we sit all afternoon…a hodgepodge of sagging livers, sinking gall bladders, drooping stomachs, compressed intestines, and squashed pelvic organs.
>
> *Dr. John Button*

Physical inactivity is rapidly being seen as a national health problem due to the detrimental effects it has on the risks of illness and disease. On a global stage, the World Health Organisation believes that physical inactivity is a major contributor in the increase of global diseases; it has become one of the major risk factors for chronic disease. It is estimated that around 60% of the world population does not achieve the recommended thirty minutes of moderate physical activity per day. Physical inactivity has been shown to increase the risks of heart disease, strokes, breast cancer, colon cancer, cardiovascular disease, diabetes, high blood pressure, obesity, and musculoskeletal problems (such as back pain and osteoporosis).

In most city communities, the environmental factors make it hard for people to incorporate physical activity into their lives. The pavements are minimised for wider roads, the roads are very busy and crossing them is a hazard in itself, cycle paths are scarce, and are often an ill thought through token gesture, with public transport systems often overcrowded, overpriced, and rarely punctual. In addition, there are problems with safety on the streets, schools, and workplaces. The workplaces are often many miles from homes, and working hours take up the most important parts of the day. Massive one-stop shopping centres are built on the outskirts of towns, where physical activity, is confined to a snails-pace walk or the use of escalators. All of these factors make staying at home or driving cars more attractive than walking or cycling.

Many industries have been built on the back of the problems arising from man's thirst for modernisation and resultant physical inactivity. For example, the health, fitness, entertainment, transport, construction, personal services, retail, energy utilities, and technology are global industries, each of which worth billions.

Most jobs now require little or no physical activity, and their home life is surrounded by new inventions, which are time-savers. This cuts the physical activity to a minimum (sometimes removing any activity completely like TV remote controls); entertainment is mostly a seated affair (television, cinema, theatre, restaurant, computer and gaming consoles, etc.), nearly everything introduced into the consumer market is 'for your convenience'; which again just reduces physical activity to the detriment of your health. The other attack comes from the abundance of food production, resulting in excess supply, overselling, and ultimately, surplus purchases. When coupled with the inferior malnourishing quality of the foods and drinks (see Part three – Nourishment), it creates an environment for overeating and superfluous excesses and a step closer to diseases, such as obesity, heart disease, high blood pressure, and diabetes.

Keep off the grass
Children are spontaneously physically active, if they have the access to appropriate facilities, or more importantly, if they are allowed to be. Children are frequently told to 'sit down', 'be still', or are being warned off communal areas, 'keep off the grass', 'no ball games'. Furthermore, with concerns for their safety, and a distinct lack of freely available areas where they can be physically active, it is no surprise that children spend more time in enclosed environments such as the home, and more often than not, are accompanied by the third parent, the television. It is not too difficult to understand then, when children are faced with these obstacles in their early years, coupled with a lack of school-based physical activity, they have been shown to be less likely to be physically active, as they grew older and into adolescence.

> In the United States, schoolchildren in grades 9 to 12,
> instead of being physically active, can be found
> watching television for at least three hours per day.

In a recent study at the University of Leicester, United Kingdom, reveals that the level of physical inactivity among children is at an epidemic scale. The researchers, Professor Kamlesh Khunti, Professor Melanie Davies, and Dr Margaret Stone, have published one of the largest studies on the physical activity levels of city schoolchildren; the study looked at over 3,500 children from five different schools. In identifying the low levels of physical activity in the schoolchildren, they highlighted the fact that half the pupils spent four hours or more a day watching television, videos or playing computer games. The parents were not any better. As even though family history of diabetes or heart disease in the parents is a risk factor, for the development of diabetes or heart disease in their children. The researchers found that the children of parents with a family history of diabetes or heart disease were just as likely to have sedentary behaviours, similar to those families without the elevated risk of disease. These are not the ideal role models.

> The American College of Sports Medicine estimated that
> five times as many Americans die from being inactive
> than from losing their lives in car accidents.

Sedentary fat gain

Physical inactivity can interfere with the body's ability to breakdown the saturated fats from the diet leading to excess body fat, and if unchecked propel a person into the health hazards associated with overweight and obesity. In the research trial, supported by the European Space Agency (Toulouse, France), a group of researchers aimed to further understand the effects of physical inactivity on the way that fat from the diet is metabolised (broken down to generate energy). Participants were randomized into two groups, both of whom underwent 90 days of bed rest, aiming to mimic sedentary behaviour. One group also received an exercise-training program during the 90 days' bed rest. The researchers examined to what extent fatty acids common in the diet were metabolized over the duration of the trial. The study showed that Resting Metabolic Rate was higher in the exercise group than the sedentary one, and it was reported that there was a physiological change in fat metabolism of one of the fatty acids, palmitate (a saturated fat). The ability of the body to breakdown the saturated fat dropped by nearly 10% in both groups. You can draw two very useful conclusions from this study, firstly, that physical activity was again proven to increase the Resting Metabolic Rate, and secondly, that just by adding a 'quick-fix' exercise training program, to an otherwise sedentary lifestyle, did not combat the detrimental physiological changes to the human body of physical inactivity. The body has a need for constant daily activity to perform at its optimum level.

The cost of doing nothing
There is also a fiscal cost of physical inactivity that is increasingly harder to ignore, this burden on the global health care system totals billions; the United States alone foots a $75 billion bill for inactivity, and coupled with obesity it costs the United States approximately 10% of total health expenditure. In a recent study conducted at the Oxford University, researchers calculated that physical inactivity was directly responsible for 3% of all United Kingdom deaths and illnesses in 2002. The researchers calculated the amount of disease and early death attributable to physical inactivity, using information from the World Health Organization. Focusing on coronary artery heart disease, stroke, breast and bowel cancers, and diabetes, they calculated the total number of deaths, illnesses, and disability associated with them. Altogether, they calculated that 287,206 people died from diseases associated with a lack of activity in 2003/4, of which more than 35,000 were directly attributable to physical inactivity. The direct cost to the United Kingdom health service, including inpatient stays, outpatient appointments, drugs, community care, and visits to primary care practitioners amounted to £1.06 billion.

All these facts and figures do not take into consideration the detrimental effect of physical inactivity on communities and economies in terms of decreased productivity, poor performing schools, higher worker absenteeism and turnover, decreased productivity and reduced participation in sports and recreational activities. In many countries, a significant proportion of health expenditure is due to costs related to lack of physical activity and obesity. Promoting physical activity can be a highly cost-effective and sustainable public health intervention.

The curse of physical inactivity can be seen at its worst when a person is immobilised. After a period of inactivity, the ability of the body tissues to utilise oxygen is noticeably reduced. In a study, participants were bed-bound and physically inactive for twenty days; and even after this very short period of inactivity, the participant's capacity to utilise oxygen was reduced by 20 to 45%. It does not stop there either, as the knock on effect is a reduction in cardiac output, muscle mass, and blood volume. Which means after just twenty days of inactivity your body is less efficient in transporting oxygen from your lungs to the tissues, and your muscles capacity to produce energy is reduced. Furthermore, the musculoskeletal system, comprising of the bones, joints, ligaments, muscles, tendons, nerves, and blood vessels, undergo qualitative changes in response to immobilisation and physical inactivity:

Bone decalcified - Bones will be weakened and will have an increased risk of suffering a fracture. The immobilisation will stimulate bone demineralisation and depress bone formation leading to osteoporosis.

Cartilage crash - The cartilage will experience water and other chemical losses; it will become soft and fragmented, the cartilage cells die, and the collagen fibres suffer irreparable damage. Extended periods of immobilisation can make the changes permanent and can lead to osteoarthritis.

Muscle wastage - Even after only one to two weeks of immobilisation your muscle mass starts to waste away. The degree of wastage depends on factors, such as duration of immobilisation, gender, and age. After a six-week period, you can expect muscle strength to diminish by 30 to 40%, its cross-sectional area by 20 to 30%, and the size of your thigh by 10 to 20%. You also lose some mechanical properties such as elasticity, and the inactive muscle structure can lead to an increased risk of joint injuries.

Tendon trouble - Tendons will also start to waste away but at a slower rate than that of muscle. The strength, elasticity, and weight of the tendon will decrease. The collagen fibres of the tendon will become thinner and disorientated. All combine to increase the risk of tendon tears and breakages.

Ligament losses - The ligament and joint capsule will become weaker. The ligament has been known to shrivel and shrink after inactivity. Total tendon mass is reduced and your mobility can be affected and excessive strains will be piled on the joints. In animal studies, ligaments have been shown to lose a quarter of their strength and elasticity. The joint capsule becomes very susceptible to overuse and irritation, and reacts by secreting excess amounts of fluid causing an overflow in the joint.

This is an example of the devastating effects of inactivity and immobilisation and the harm it can cause to your physical wellness. It is never too late to start rehabilitation from these negative effects of physical inactivity.

Chapter 17

Activity for life

Physical activity is a fundamental component of good health and well-being, and by adding regular bouts of activity to your daily routine, it will bring many benefits that increase the quality of your life. Physical activities do not need to be overly strenuous for a person to enjoy benefits to health; in fact, only a moderate level of activity is required to get most of the health benefits available.

It benefits people of all ages and is often more fun when done with friends or family. Being active with parents or grandparents is not just a great way to stay healthy, but it can be a time to bond with loved ones. Knowing that regular physical activity offers great benefits to all ages is a good reason to make physical activity a family affair.

> Thinking well is wise; planning well, wiser; doing well, wisest of them all.
>
> *Persian proverb*

Healthy living and physical activity are inseparably linked; physical activity is an essential part of being able to lead a healthy long life. It is never too late to start being more physically active and reap its growing list of benefits.

According to the World Health Organisation, regular physical activity will:

- reduce the risk
  - of dying prematurely
  - of dying from heart disease or stroke
  - of developing heart disease or colon cancer by up to 50%
  - of developing type 2 diabetes by 50%
  - of developing lower back pain
- help to prevent / reduce

o hypertension
o osteoporosis, reducing the risk of hip fracture by up to 50% in women
- promote psychological well-being, reduces stress, anxiety and feelings of depression and loneliness
- help prevent or control risky behaviours, especially among children and young people, like tobacco, alcohol or other substance use, unhealthy diet or violence
- help control weight and lower the risk of becoming obese by 50% compared to people with sedentary lifestyles
- help build and maintain healthy bones, muscles, and joints and makes people with chronic, disabling conditions improve their stamina
- help in the management of painful conditions, like back pain or knee pain

A healthy heart

Regular physical activity makes for a healthier heart. There is no organ more important than the heart; a strong and efficient heart is able to supply the brain and the rest of the body with a fresh supply of oxygenated blood, while also clearing out the toxic waste products. How well the heart performs is a good indication of how healthy the cardiovascular (the heart and the blood vessels) system is. A healthy level of cardiovascular fitness will give you the ability to continue to do a stressful activity, such as brisk walking, running, heavy gardening, and riding a bike, for an extended period of time and will also allow you to return to your normal heart and breathing rate more quickly afterwards. In short, a healthy and efficient heart and lungs supplies oxygenated blood and therefore, more fuel to be used for energy, to your muscles, which then increases your body's capacity to display a higher level of effort.

> As people grow older, their lung capacity or how much
> air the lungs hold, grows smaller
>
> *Health-Warrior*

By gradually elevating your levels of physical activity, you will strengthen your heart and lungs and improve your blood circulation. As physical activity uses your body's largest muscles groups (the legs), it will increase your oxygen requirements, and if maintained over a period of time (weeks, months, and years) it will improve the functioning and efficiency of your heart and lungs. Furthermore, it will make it easier to perform everyday functional and purposeful activities such as climbing stairs, mowing the lawn, and carrying groceries.

What should you do? All children and adults should aim to achieve at least thirty minutes of moderate-intensity activity every day of the week. It is easier to incorporate moderate intensity activity into your life, as it covers a wide variety of normal daily activities, and can be tailored to an individual's needs, preferences, and life circumstances. Moreover, to make things even easier to adhere to and complete, the thirty minutes of time can be accumulated through segments of at least ten minutes.

You can use physical activity to lose weight and/or maintain a healthy weight; the thirty minutes per day of moderate intensity activity (though you may need to increase your intensity gradually) will help you as long as you are careful about how much you eat (see Part three - Nourishment). A report from the Institute of Medicine concluded that daily moderate-intensity activity is useful to maintain a healthy weight. Among the 3,000 men and women who are part of the National Weight Control Registry, a select club that includes only people who lost more than thirty pounds and kept them off for at least a year, the average participant burns an average of 400 calories per day in physical activity. That is the equivalent of about an hour of brisk walking.

Moderate intensity physical activity will cause a slight but noticeable increase in breathing and heart rate; the physical activity should be hard enough to break into a sweat but also comfortable enough to carry on a conversation. For example, brisk walking as if late for an important appointment should be enough for most people.

In fact, walking is a perfect activity, not requiring any special equipment, can be done anytime and anywhere, and is very safe for the general population. It is what we are built to do. It is also a great way to burn fat; after thirty minutes of sustained brisk walking you will start to burn 50% glycogen and more importantly 50% fat (whereas the higher the intensity of exercise your body will use up more glycogen instead of fat). A brisk daily walk of thirty minutes or more will burn higher levels of fat than the torture people go through at the gym in the equivalent time.

When trying to promote physical activity, you can often hear me say things like 'energy creates energy' or 'laziness is energy wasted'. As everything you do requires energy; so you would think that, a physically active person would have less energy than someone who is inactive. This is not the case, and could not be further from the truth, as a person who engages in physical activity will display an increased level of energy (as well as an increased capacity) throughout the entire day, while the inactive person will be lethargic and report tiredness (due to their decreased and decreasing capacity) in the same period. This capacity comes from your ability to process oxygen within a specific period of time, also known as your aerobic capacity; the greater your aerobic capacity, the greater your energy levels.

This increased vitality means you can take in large quantities of the oxygen into your bloodstream and deliver it more efficiently to its cells and tissues; giving a big boost to body functions such as, your immune system, which helps fight colds, illnesses and diseases, and speeds up recovery from all kinds of injuries. The less time a person is ill, the more energy a person has to spend on living well. On the other hand, a sedentary person will not be able to pump as much oxygen around their body in a similar about of time; and suffer from a poor immune system, consequently, having a weaker ability to fight off illness or disease, and less time to enjoy life.

In addition, to physical activity, people should engage in strength training and flexibility and stability sessions at least twice a week, which will promote the maintenance of lean body mass, improvements in muscular strength and endurance, and preservation of body function, all of which enable long-term participation in regular physical activity and promote quality of life.

Daily strength

The muscles of your body are under constant pressure to resist force; it is this ability to resist force, which represents your body strength. Regular physical activity builds strength and endurance in your muscles; similar to the improvements made in your heart and lungs, allowing you to perform activities more easily, such as carrying groceries, lifting heavy objects, digging in the garden, or moving furniture. Strength training is probably the most neglected component of your health and well-being, but is one of the most beneficial. Muscle is full of 'calorie-burning machines' and it utilises the calories to perform work, and to repair and refuel itself. Body fat, on the other hand, has no such machines and just hangs around burning very few calories.

From the late twenties onwards, you start to lose muscle as part of your natural aging process. This means you start to lose calorie-burning machines too, and therefore, do not burn as many calories as the day before, making it easier to gain weight. Strength training will maintain and sometimes increase or replace the number of these machines. Studies have shown strength-training adaptations can increase lean body mass, decrease fat mass, and increase Resting Metabolic Rate (a basic measurement of the amount of calories you burn per day). These three very important factors empower you to maintain and manage a healthy weight. An efficient and strong body will help you in maintaining a leaner and healthier body.

A body, which has inadequate muscle strength, will reduce the quality of life in that person as they age. Moreover, at the other end of the spectrum, a body, which is overly muscular and strong in relation to its shape and structure, can put an unnecessary pressure on vital functions and organs of the body, increase the risks of injury, reduce flexibility, and restrict ranges of movement. The key is to promote strength and endurance in your muscles with a variety of regular weight-bearing activities, such as walking, climbing stairs, carrying a backpack or groceries, and gardening. These types of activities if performed on a regular basis will help build stronger bones in the areas affected by the activity being done; for example, walking will promote strength in the bones of your legs, and the carrying of groceries, the bones of your arm, back, and legs.

It is important here to add that you do not have to belong to a gym or have a house full of free-weights in order to perform weight-bearing activities and gain the rewards. As, not only will the varieties of weight-bearing physical activity in daily living build stronger muscles, promote stronger bones, and healthy joints; it will also improve balance, stability, and coordination.

The older you get, the need for strength training increases, as it can help maintain the ability to perform basic functional tasks such as walking, rising from a chair, climbing stairs, carrying groceries, as well as help prevent the risk of falls and injuries. More importantly, regular strength training in older adults will also help combat debilitating diseases, such as arthritis, a disease that involves the chronic inflammation of the joints, and osteoporosis, one that gradually weakens bones, making them so fragile that they can fracture easily while performing everyday activities. A disease such as osteoporosis does not happen overnight and takes years to develop, with many people unaware that they have the disease until it is too late. It is common for a person to only find out they have the disease after they suffer a bone fracture; the results are painful and can go on to be an irreversible crippling condition. For example, in postmenopausal women, two strength-training sessions a week for one year increased bone mineral density by 1%. While a sedentary control group lost 2% in the same time.

Flexibility and stability
It used to be the case that young people were quite flexible but even this is beginning to change, as more and more children are reported as being inadequately physically active. This can be a worrying situation, as the population ages, as with heart and lung capacity, flexibility diminishes with age. Flexibility and stability are two components of overall physical fitness and should be actively worked on everyday.

Flexibility is the ability to move a joint painlessly through its full range of motion and will contribute to a continued quality of living and reduce the risks of injury as a person ages. The static stretching of a muscles and joints is an effective and popular technique to ensure continued functional ranges of motion. Sitting on the floor with your legs outstretched in front of you while reaching smoothly forward to touch (or try to) your toes is a good example of static stretching. It is also suggested that maintaining normal ranges of joint and muscle flexibility can help prevent back pain and osteoarthritis.

Stability can encompass agility, balance, coordination, and speed of movement, and is important at all stages of life to maintain independence and a high quality of living. It is especially important during growth and as an older adult. As children there is a need to develop basic motor skills to help secure optimum future physical wellness; and as older adults there is a need to 'relearn' these components of stability to help prevent falls, avoid accidents, and preserve independence and live a quality of life to which a person has become accustomed to.

Walking on grassy fields, a beach, uneven ground, playing with children, or attending yoga or T'ai chi sessions are examples of disciplines where people can work on, among other things, increasing flexibility and stability.

The physical activity and mental health

Physical activity is beneficial to the mind as well as the body; to achieve these benefits for your mental health, a person should do something active everyday of the week. The great thing about physical activity is that it does not matter what a person does as long as it raises the heart rate for a certain period of time (even accumulative activity durations of ten minutes will do); it is something you enjoy; and it is safe and is purposeful.

Improve concentration and memory

Concentration is important for learning and understanding new things and being able to perform well in all aspects of life. Being physically active can help improve concentration. This means, that a person will be able to be more focused and perform better. Staying physically fit has also been found to help people maintain memory longer in their lives. As people get older, their memory skills can deteriorate, and physical activity can help ward off this effect for some time.

Stress-busters

Stress is a normal part of every person's life. It is actually necessary to have some stress in life, as life without stress would be unsafe. However, too much stress can cause many health problems. Chronic stress can increase your risk of conditions such as heart disease, high blood pressure, a suppressed immune system, eating disorders, headaches, sleep disorders, and ulcers.

In Robert Sapolsky's excellent book on stress, 'Why zebras don't get ulcers', he takes you on an expertly simplified journey through the complicated maze of physiological responses and reactions to stress. According to Sapolsky, stress can disrupt and reduce many physiological functions such as:

- Digestion; increasing risks of ulcers, and reducing nutrient uptake, and appetite
- Long term memory; increasing neuron damage
- metabolism; increasing in fatigue, inefficiency, muscle atrophy, and risks of diabetes
- Reproduction; reducing sexual function
- Growth; decreasing growth hormone, nutrients, and increasing growth inhibitors and bone problems
- Immune system; reducing protection and increasing susceptibility to disease
- Aging; increasing rate of aging, decreasing life expectancy, and increasing risks of mental illness
- Pain responses; desensitises the sensors which detect pain

Physical activities, especially non-competitive ones, help to manage stress; though will not eliminate the sources of the stress. If performed regularly it can offset the negative stress emotions (such as anger, fear, and sadness) and enhance positive stress emotions (such as love, joy, and surprise).

Physical activity and mental health continued
Mental health is a serious public health issue, and in a study commissioned by the World Health Organisation and the World Bank it indicated that four out of every ten leading causes of disability for persons aged five and over, are mental disorders, such as depression, manic-depressive, schizophrenia, and obsessive-compulsive. The World Health Organisation estimates that by the year 2020, depression will surpass cancer as the second leading worldwide cause of disability and death (behind cardiovascular disease). There are many studies, which support the fact that physical activity can decrease anxiety, prevent and reduce the incidence of mild and moderate depression, and improve self-esteem.

Dampening depression

Major depression is a common health disorder with serious effects. Treatments can be time-consuming and medications can be highly addictive with unsavoury side effects. Physical activity has been used to combat the effects of depression as long ago as 500BC; Hippocrates prescribed physical activity to those with melancholic symptoms. So it comes as little surprise that recent studies indicate that physical activity can reduce the primary risks of depression and can alleviate the symptoms from suffers of mild to moderate depression.

Putting the 'self' back into self-esteem

The physical self, which includes the physical body, is an important part of self-esteem, more so in Western societies with increasing influence in developing ones. Physical activity can improve the self-esteem for most people, but especially those who display the lowest measures of it, with psychosocial factors such as, improved perceptions of competence or appearance, mobility independence, and sense of well-being. In recent studies, it was shown that almost 80% of them showed significant changes in self-worth and other self-perceptions after physical activity.

Anti-anxiety

Anxiety is a state of worry, apprehension, or tension that often occurs in the sense of real or obvious danger; it becomes a disorder when the symptoms or behaviours are frequent and severe, causing impairment of the normal physical and social function. Common anxiety disorders include phobias, panic attacks, obsessive-compulsive behaviours, and posttraumatic stress. Physical activity has been shown to reduce levels of anxiety. In a study, which examined the effects of physical activity and patients with various anxiety disorders, it was reported that after an eight-week period of activity (three one-hour sessions per week) all participants showed reductions in anxiety.

Your physical activity action plan

To summarise, physical activity is something you are born to do; it is part of your genetic make-up, where the mechanics of which have evolved over millions of years, with your basic genes remaining unchanged for the last 10,000 years or so. To be physically active is of great importance in your quest for health, well-being, quality of life, and longevity in this modern age, as it was back in the Stone Age, in promoting the optimal human performance ensuring an efficient body function, and producing reductions in the risk of both physical and mental illness and disease.

By making small changes in your lifestyle, you can enjoy the big changes of better health. Paraphrasing a popular quote by Lord

Chesterfield makes the point perfectly, 'take care of the activity minutes, for the activity hours will take care of themselves'. In addition, you should avoid giving yourself 'body beautiful' or aesthetic goals; your goals should only revolve around trying to improve your health.

The perfect size of a body is a healthy one.

Health-Warrior

How do you make physical activity a permanent part of your life?

1. Make it enjoyable and purposeful; will mean you are more likely to stick to it
2. Make it social and seek support; a friend, colleagues, a partner, children can introduce 'activity' time to your moments of quality time
3. Integrate physical activity into your present lifestyle and preferences; to increase your physical activity opportunities
4. Reward yourself; set yourself a motivating targets and once you achieve it enjoy your reward

What should you do?

1. Brisk walking for at least thirty minutes per day (or an equivalent type of moderate physical activity
2. Perform strength training activities
3. Continually seek to maintain or improve your flexibility and stability

Some ideas to add extra amounts of physical activity to your life:

- Walk and cycle whenever you can as transport
- Use the stairs or walk the escalators whenever possible
- Use public transport; walk up or down the escalators, get off a stop earlier and walk the remaining distance
- Find local hills, stairs, open spaces to vary your walking activity
- At every opportunity walk instead of standing; stand instead of sitting; sit instead of lying down
- If you have to use your car (try to car share); and if safe, park further away and walk
- Shop locally; spread grocery purchases over the week; it means more frequent visits, fresher foods, and also increases your strength training
- Take up gardening, even if it is growing herbs in a window basket

- Do something around the house daily; for example, DIY or housework
- Try to do household chores manually; dusting, polishing, sweeping, mopping, etc; (a clean house is a healthy one)
- Play with children
- Dance (no rhythm or ability to dance required! Let the music play and go for it; behind closed doors if you have to)
- Play an instrument

Personal Care:
- Shower and towel dry with vigorous and fast movements
- Stand when grooming (e.g. washing face, shaving, brushing teeth, etc.)
- Stand on alternating feet while grooming (works on your stability and balance)
- Use different hands grooming (e.g. use left hand instead of right for brushing teeth: works new muscles and helps with coordination)
- Dress and undress while standing

Work:

- Use work lunch hours for activity
- Go for walking meetings, instead of say, the unhealthy 'working lunch'
- Introduce standing meetings; after removing tables and chairs from meeting rooms
- Stand while performing tasks (where possible); such as making or returning phone calls, and opening and reading mail
- Take regular breaks away from your desk
- Perform stretching movements at your desk

Watch out for and try to avoid physical activity killers:
- Time constraints; such as not having time to be active due to overworking;
- Watching TV, remote controls, computer use, gaming consoles, films, internet shopping, home delivery services, riding in a car or train, DIY power tools, kitchen gadgets, cordless phones, etc.;
- Excessive reading of newspapers, magazines, books, etc.

Part six

A silent revolution

This book has focused mostly on the essential human needs: oxygen, water, nourishment, sleep, and physical activity. Each of these sections has shown that people are railroaded into the living excess, indulgence, extravagance, or covetous lifestyles, creating serious concerns and problems for the future of human health. It is simplicity of living and lifestyle moderation, which will lead you to fulfilment, happiness, and a higher quality of life.

Simplicity of living is a conscious choice and effort to perform a reality-check and appraisal of all your wants and desires, in relation to your essential needs. It is one where artificial 'necessities' of life are unceremoniously discarded if they do not add something meaningful and measurable to your quality of life. It is time to take a look at the battleground where the future of your health will be fought, and won or lost.

The battle for health
In compiling the Health-Warrior, it was evident that there are many intertwined factors and forces, which effect good health and well-being. No one factor or force stood above the others in importance. Nevertheless, my personal research, feedback from clients, and the studies of others pointed me to the fact that most of the forces of ill health stem from the movement and continual renewal of what is referred to as 'modernisation'. The genetics of a person may seem like an obvious exclusion, however I suspect that in the future that even the genes of a person will be shown as being affected by modernisation.

Having lived in London through five decades, I am in an advantageous position to comment on one of the key players and undisputed hubs of the modernisation movement: the continually expanding global cities. The cities have set their sights on everything green, the open green pastures and woodlands, clearing over half of the world's original forest cover and leaving 30% of the rest degraded or fragmented, as well as the 'greenback', money. Its continued development is visible to most, such as the unstoppable expanding web of transportation, the endless streams of trains, planes, cars, buses, coaches, and trucks, and the seemingly permanent road works and building sites that are fuelled by the continual need of, for example, more transportation routes, power and energy supplies, housing, and commercial premises. People strive for modernisation at every juncture and no one appears to be able to stand in the way of this seemingly ceaseless advance toward infinite profit and prosperity. Modernisation, for me, is the pursuit of convenience and extravagance and is the driving force behind the expansion of concrete and its unquestionable ability to bury life underneath it.

> Two thirds of Earth is covered by a blue sea, and the
> remaining third a blueprint for a city.
>
> *Health-Warrior*

A growing pressure for expansion comes about from the expanding population and the constant migration of people to the cities. Why is it that all roads seem to lead to the city? What takes people there? Alternatively, for those born there, what stops them from leaving? Preying on instinctual human greed, the city is a place where people are lured to with tales of profit and prosperity. However, it seemed to me that the promise of 'only available in the city' riches, was built on the foundations of the prefabricated 'desires' of a person and their perceived need for success or their fear of failure. The stream of people to the city resembles the tune that the Pied Piper played while luring the children away from their family and home.

The tale of profit and prosperity was so great that the first generation of migrants were heard to complain that the city was not actually paved with gold, and money did not grow on the trees. The lure and its promises, I noticed had become much more than just about the perceived level of success or failure or indeed money. The city promised affiliation to the 'City Club', a move away from an 'underdeveloped' village or countryside scene, and offered a comforting level of social or peer approval. Humans are seen as social creatures, and as such, much of their satisfaction comes from other people. To a point, people need other people to sustain a whole life of health and well-being, one where family and friends provide loving, caring, and nurturing relationships. However, observing the changes about me, I began to doubt the extent to which people derived their satisfaction from random contact with other people. City living has demanded that people are stacked one on top of the other, stacked high, as they are wide, which seems to create more aggravation, frustration, and irritation than satisfaction from constant contact with other people. There is no sign of community, families and friends can be widely dispersed about the globe, and neighbours just anonymous faces. In fact, a collection of books, stacked high, and wide in a library has more community than most streets of a city.

London, the city, produces very little for itself and relatively nothing in the case of farming and agriculture. It is a city, which cannot supply its own needs and instead it has to rely on others. It consumes copious amounts of resources and energy from the Earth's limited and diminishing natural supplies. This reliance on others has been regularly reducing the world's cropland since the 1950's. As the population of London increased, so did its need for more construction, and consumption. The one visible consequence of the 'success' of London was the excessive amounts of pollution and waste materials.

As I visited other major cities of the world, the picture was no different and I consequently took more of an interest in how the environment was being eroded and polluted on a daily basis, and just as important, how this pollution was influencing a person's health and well-being. The raw materials and natural resources, that modernisation has become so heavily dependant on, have started to show signs of diminishing supplies. Increasing global consumption places a huge burden on finding new resources and the subsequent waste management. Road traffic and industrial air pollution brought new meaning to the 'grey' days in London, and it was another sprawling metropolis stateside, which introduced people to the new word 'smog'. An increasing number of people seemed to be adversely affected by the reducing air quality, and more of my client base, displayed respiratory and breathing difficulties in their daily lives.

Clean water is something I grew up with and took for granted, which I can forcefully say is not the case today. The demand for water has tripled globally in the last fifty years. The water supplies of today are becoming increasingly scarce, and it is predicted that people living in water stressed or scarce countries will increase by 400 to 600% or 2.4 to 3.4 billion by 2025. In addition, of the sources, which are available, show signs of increased pollution, with pollutants, such as inadequately treated sewage, fertilisers, silt, oil, petroleum, waste materials, microscopic waterborne chemicals, and pesticides, which in turn are guilty of transporting many illnesses into people's lives with an ever-increasing efficiency.

Food and drink supplies appear to be unaffected by the increasing numbers of people or the expanding needs of the city, as they appear to be unlimited in quantity and variety. However, on closer inspection, food and drink is just as polluted and influenced by the expanding numbers of people and the inability of the city to produce its own resources. 'Real' food, as it is found in nature, is actually decreasing in supply, relative to the 'unreal' processed and packaged kind. The local convenience store may have a few unnaturally produced apples or oranges (their token gesture of real food), but the majority of the store is filled with the packaged and processed varieties that have days, weeks, or years, worth of shelf life. As with any form of pollution exposure, the short-term effect can be illness and the longer-term one a cause of disease.

While on my travels, I learned firsthand about how the lack of quality sleep can be a silent and detrimental influencer of human health and well-being. While flying from one country to another across multiple time zones, I would be adversely affected by the disruption to my sleep. After a flight, I could only manage a few hours of sleep, after which would be pestered by an unnatural fatigue and a dull headache. It would take me at least twenty-four hours to adjust and return to a less damaging sleep pattern. After a person's need for quality supplies of air, water, and food, sleep is the next most important factor in achieving better health. In an urban setting, the factors influencing the disruption of sleep are many, such as noise and light pollution, stress and anxiety, excessive stimulation, poor nutrition, and long working hours. The working hours of a city are twenty-four hours long and operate on a seven-day a week basis, and this, 'open-for-business at all hours', increases sleep related problems and illnesses. My previous working routines, when I was less attentive and blind to my health needs, would start at 4.45am and finish at 10pm, with my first client at 6am and the last at 9pm. I would barely manage five hours sleep and the eventual outcome would be a mental or physical fall of some kind, and it could appear as displays of frustration or as minor ailments such as headaches or body aches. Sleep is so important that it is not an area to be toyed with; a person should spend a third of their lives enjoying the revitalising and rejuvenating benefits of sleep.

Another consequence, of the expanding city, is the reduced opportunities to interact with nature and partake in physical activity, which are both vital to better health and well-being. Humans are supposed to be born into nature and are built to walk, yet with every modern step and the arrival of yet more concrete and asphalt; they are being taken for a ride further away from their natural habitat, and deprived of places to walk due to the increases in urbanisation. Although, Central London, had a few beautiful parks and green spaces (a legacy of a rich history and monarchy), it still suffered miserably with masses of traffic packed roads and a 'concrete jungle' habitat. It supplies few outside areas for physical activity relative to the number of people who live there, and the amount of space afforded to the car.

The foundations of vitality and a healthier lifestyle it seems are slowly slipping from the clasps of people, similar to what would happen if you tried to grab and hold handfuls of sand without spilling any. What could distract people so much, that they would relinquish their health and well-being for it?

The constant sale
On an average working day, I would be confronted with over five hundred advertisements in some shape or form. The city is a primary source of proliferation of this kind of lifestyle propaganda, of which advertisements are a major part, using multiple media sources such as television, radio, internet, mail, posters, books, magazines, newspapers, and other people to get their message across. The lifestyle messages are pushed and peddled by among others, governments, industries, companies, media, experts, specialists, and peer groups, which has made the journey toward a better life, a battle of attrition, instead of one of adventure and discovery. It is a fight for, which a person needs to have a strategy for living, and a way to defend themselves from the constant battering. Losing the battle will represent a high price to pay, monetary as well as physically and emotionally. These direct, indirect, or subliminal messages are aimed at a person's psychological and emotional instincts. These selling techniques seek to reward, comfort, and pacify a person, in response to the prefabricated discontent and a host of perceived needs, which the lifestyle propaganda generates.

Everyday was a meeting with abundance, extravagance, and convenience with which I could access many of the so-called 'good' things of life. Over zealous consumerism on the back of excess production and overselling, seems to be the driving force behind most of the global economies, with a portion of the world's people trying to produce something to sell, another portion devoted to persuading people they need it, and the last portion dedicated to accumulating as much enjoyment from the purchase process and the products as they can. Are they truly the good things in life? Do they produce moments of true enjoyment or satisfaction?

People are inundated with new products and services, preceded by waves of emotional and psychological advertising and marketing of all kinds. This enormous pressure to adopt a newer standard of living on a every wakeful hour seems to be based solely on the maintenance of a prosperous economy and has little regard for the physical and mental health of people in that economy or elsewhere. People are being repeatedly sold the idea that continual modernisation and new technology can, and will have the ability to solve all their worldly and spiritual problems. This kind of blind faith appears to push a person unconsciously further into the claws of superfluous and mindless consumption.

Can too much of anything be a good thing?
Who does not want to consume foods that are more delicious and easier to prepare, want to do more stimulating things, or seek objects of greater expense and rarity? What I would observe around me were people with insatiable desires for all things 'new' in copious quantities, never happy with what they had, and always one-step behind where they wanted to be. The insatiable desire was fuelled by the lifestyle propaganda machine, and it was creating and maintaining a constant gap between their perceived needs and their present situation, a formula for successful consumerism.

I noticed that people would not question the origins or the reasons behind the messages cajoling them into a state of prefabricated discontent. The 'discontent', would move people in different ways but it usually ended with a person's constant and uncultivable need for 'amusement'. This need for amusement or mood modifier was catered for via consumption; the opportunity for people to 'buy, buy, buy', any product or service in order to acquire positive feelings, increases in self-worth, status, satisfaction leading to what they would see as social approval and affiliation of some kind.

In response to this a person would spend most of their free time, either consuming these messages of their 'unhappiness' and 'inadequate' standard of current living, or in the active pursuit of products or services, which they thought would make them happier or less inadequate. Such amusement and the perceived associations of increased self-worth, status, satisfaction, and standard of living seemed to be directly related to the number of amusement experiences and value of money spent. The more amusement experiences encountered and the more money spent on them, the greater the perceived self-worth, status, satisfaction, and standard of living would be.

Will you ever truly be happy by spending (or borrowing to spend) the hard-earned cash that you work for, on products or service which somebody else tells you that you need? Given this situation it was no surprise to me, that one of the hazards of this kind of lifestyle, which was confined within the walls of modernisation and consumerism, led to people around me who were psychologically and physically ailing, and always seeking something more fulfilling from life but in reality moving further away from it.

It seems to me as though the consumerism of today is much different from the materialism, of the eighties for example, where the economic boom in the some countries and the apparent abundance of money, saw people buy for the sake of buying to accumulate as many material goods as they could. The difference in the last twenty years or so has seen a new breed of consumer come to life, who is much more interested in the act of consumption and the positive emotions they elicit, rather than the accumulation of material goods. For those who are waiting for consumerism to crash or implode my prediction is that they will be waiting a long time. Whereas in previous decadent and hedonistic societies, the elite classes were eventually overthrown by the masses, and a return to some sort of people parity was assumed, the consumerism of today is so unabatedly successful because it is the 'masses' who are the driving force at the centre of the pursuit of these perceived pleasures and amusements in life.

When will the average person get bored of their numerous playthings and amusements, casting them aside for the sake of a better and healthier life? Will there ever be a time when the boredom and despair of a society be able to free itself of the attachment to consumption?

Creating the need

Industries, the food industry a good example, has been built and profitably maintained by this type of health and lifestyle propaganda. The powerful food industry is constantly advising, consulting, cajoling, persuading, and pressuring the consumer into making purchases that are taking them further away from their goal of optimum health, happiness, and fulfilment.

A supermarket, close to where I used to live in London, would be open 24hrs a day and would sit on a plot of land the size of five football fields. It would stock thousands of food and drink items per isle and tens of thousands per store that were piled high and sold cheap (or not so cheap), without any concern for a person's health and well-being. They continue to ignore the fact that over consumption of the highly processed, additive-laden, and unreal foods and drinks on sale continue to be associated as major contributing factors to illness and death in society today, costing millions financially, and immeasurable emotional and physical pain. Moreover, there was an almost zero percent chance of choosing a product on sale that could claim to be seasonal, ethically and locally farmed/produced, free of additives, chemicals, and genetic modification, and be a genuinely 'as it is found in nature' food or drink.

My nutrition consultations revolved around empowering people to source 'real' foods, which are the best suppliers of the nutrients for good health, from their local farmers markets and other similar sources. Moreover, if they had to shop at a supermarket, my advice was to visit the one isle of real food, the fruit, and vegetables one, which was always the first isle in the supermarket, buy the locally sourced organic marked items, and proceed to the checkout. The choices available in a supermarket will always be much greater than the ones available through local farming sources, as the farmers find it near impossible to compete with the buying power and economies of scale of supermarket giants. However, the seemingly expansive choices at the supermarket carries many items of food and drinks, which contributes to a person's increased risk of ill health, and one where these choices of packaged, processed, additive-laden, and unreal foods were also guilty of introducing people to varieties of allergies, hypersensitivities, addictions and intolerances.

Passing the buck
Not so surprisingly to me was the fact that most of the 'cures' for such ailments arising from malnourishing foods could be found in the highly lucrative medical, biotechnological, chemical, health, and alternative health industries. There is seemingly an operation, test, therapy, drug, potion, lotion, supplement pill, or powder for every current human suffering, and there is, an adequately qualified surgeon, consultant, doctor, therapist, expert, or specialist, who is more than ready and willing to administer them. This powerful industry owes much of its success to the malfunctioning city, producing malfunctioning people. It is an industry, which produces its own very powerful lifestyle propaganda to sell 'health' and is accused of disease mongering in many situations. Just looking at the recent balance sheets of the top 10 United States pharmaceutical companies, their expenditures for marketing (and a little on administration) were 31% of sales, which accounted for an amazing $67 billion of their $217 billion in sales.

> Spending in the United States for prescription drugs was $179.2 billion in 2003, almost 4½ times larger than the $40.3 billion spent in 1990.
> *Source: US National Health Accounts*

'Don't do drugs' was a message that was aimed predominantly at young people who were tempted by the use of drugs such as ecstasy, cannabis, cocaine, and heroin (their consumption can be seen as behaviours searching for constant amusement). However, I was always left with the thoughts that the drug awareness campaign should have been directed at the wider population who habitually use, often leading to addiction and problematic withdrawal symptoms, the drugs such as sleeping pills, anti-depressants, and painkillers prescribed or taken under advice. No drug or treatment will completely cure any illness or disease, without sending the body out of balance (and into potential danger) elsewhere. The people around me mostly fell into three categories: serial drug and treatment users (prescribed or personal purchases); occasional user (as and when symptoms arose); those who would avoid all forms of drugs or treatments. The pharmaceutical industry will actively target the occasional users, as here are the potential new 'serial' ones; targeting the serial users or the avoid-all-drugs groups would show little return on their advertising and marketing investment.

A healthy population requires a no need for drugs, whereas an unhealthy one requires more drugs and treatments. Increased drug sales provide the cash for more research, and more research amounts to newer drugs and treatments, more drugs and treatments use marketing and advertising to promise less ill or disease-ridden people, and therefore, increase drug sales. Catering for the pharmaceutical needs of people suffering from illness or disease is a very lucrative business, with the likes of Pfizer, the world's number-one drug company, boasting a profit margin of 26% of sales. The pharmaceutical industry's profits continue to be around 14% of sales, which is extraordinary when you compare it to the median of 4.6% for other industries. Extraordinary profits point unequivocally to excessively high prices.

However, for me the lucrative industry of illness and disease, underplays the risks of using drugs, preying on the hope and despair of people, while overemphasising their benefits. Drugs for diseases such as cancer are routinely rushed into use, even though the treatments are unproven and often rely on clinical trials, which have not completed their term. These experimental treatments are then unleashed on desperate patients and mostly given no other choice but to participate. These people are already suffering enough with a disease like cancer; do they really have to endure the experiments of overzealous doctors (supported by the pharmaceutical companies)?

Are there any drugs available, which deliver real cures, ones that would remove the symptoms of the illness or disease without causing some kind of internal damage elsewhere?

On the other hand, why does it seem like your local doctor or chemist is intent on supplying you with any drug or treatment, which comes closest to your symptoms, instead of addressing the cause? It may be because the education of medical students and doctors in the use of prescription drugs is funded and supported by drug companies, in the shape of seminars, conferences, meetings, and printed educational ('sales') materials. The billions spent on this 'education', as well as incentives, presents and other blandishments, comes out of the marketing budget of the pharmaceutical companies.

A government should be protecting its citizens from dangerous situations like this. However, in fact it seems to add fuel to the fire. Since 2003, the UK Government has been heavily promoting self-medication through a number of initiatives, such as a health information strategy, expert patient, walk-in centres, pharmacy-centred advice, as well as through legislation, public education and the restructuring of the National Health Service. In addition, it introduced a streamlined delisting process to facilitate the entry of new products, while a relaxation of regulations has permitted a greater variety of retail outlets to sell such products (such as supermarkets). The effect provided an improved access to the powerful prescription-only drugs for the public, and resulted in approximately £2.1bn of over-the-counter pharmaceuticals retail sales in 2005.

Passing the buck...again
One of the consequences I noted of a tampered body balance was the creation of another illness or disease, due to factors such as the consumption of malnourishing foods or the use of drugs and treatments. Most of the overweight and obese people I consulted would fall into to one of the two factors above. The solutions put forward for tackling overweight and obese people, conveniently ignored the masses of malnourishing foods and the effects of drug and treatment use, to focus on a less controversial aspect, exercise. The last twenty years has seen the sedentary person as the guilty one, and the reason behind the increases of all modern illnesses and diseases. The propaganda push established a rapidly growing health and fitness industry to cater for the exercise needs of people. Gyms, fitness centres, and health clubs were seen as the 'new hope' in the battle against illness and disease; and this continues to be the case. However, the human only needs to be moderately physically active for optimum health and well-being. There is no need for the mountains of exercise equipment, classes, and activities on offer at these types of establishments, when a daily brisk walk for thirty minutes is enough for most people.

The problems are created for instance, when people are bombarded with messages to consume malnourishing foods and drinks, which they consume, and in increasing quantities in order to attain the body's vitamin and mineral requirements. The increased consumption of excessive calories leads to excess body fat (if unchecked, leading to obesity and its health risks). Propaganda from (your Government for example) chastises people for consuming the detrimental foods or drinks, without actually addressing the sales of them, and promotes exercise as the 'ideal choice' to rectify the problem. Again, the real causes of the illness or disease are not addressed. Moreover, excessive exercise to try to rectify over consumption of inadequately nourishing foods is just further adding to the stresses upon the body, leading to future body malfunctions and the creation of new ailments.

The only solution
Simplicity of living is your conscious choice to fight back and recover your health and well-being, depress all your frivolous wants and desires, and focus on your essential needs. If what you say, think, or do does not add something meaningful and measurable to your quality of life, then it is time to reject it and live a life which is 'simply the best'.

Chapter 18

The power of simple living

Simple living is the ultimate goal for people seeking the power of moderation and balance, and will provide a greater focus and concentration on the living essentials and therefore, create an increased quality of life. It is a conscious move towards the accumulation of health and well-being, as oppose to the accumulation of wealth and amusements. This deliberate choice for a person is one that is the marriage of their ideals and integrity.

> When you arise in the morning, think what a precious privilege it is to live, to breathe, to think, to enjoy, to love.
>
> *Marcus Aurelius*

The art of simple living encompasses the most essential needs for human existence:

- Oxygen, water, nourishment, sleep, and physical activity
- Shelter and warmth; protection from the elements
- Social contact; family, friends, and community
- Freedom; the liberty and means to pursue the above

Ideally, simple living is a question of balance and moderation, and all human action should sit comfortably in the moderation band (see table on the next page). It is to be expected that there will be occasions where a person will slip out of this band, and experience excess, indulgence, extravagance, or covetous behaviours. Nevertheless, as long as the majority of activity takes place in the moderation band it will be a pathway to a healthier life. Incidentally, in developed and developing countries, it will be rare though not impossible, for a person to experience the other end of the spectrum: deficiency and depravation.

To live a life within the moderation band will require many attributes, such as courage, mental strength, and optimism. However, it is discipline, which will be the essential attribute guiding you to success, and ultimately your freedom; it makes it possible for you to reach just about any goal in your life, with the first goal of every person being (or should be) the attainment of better health.

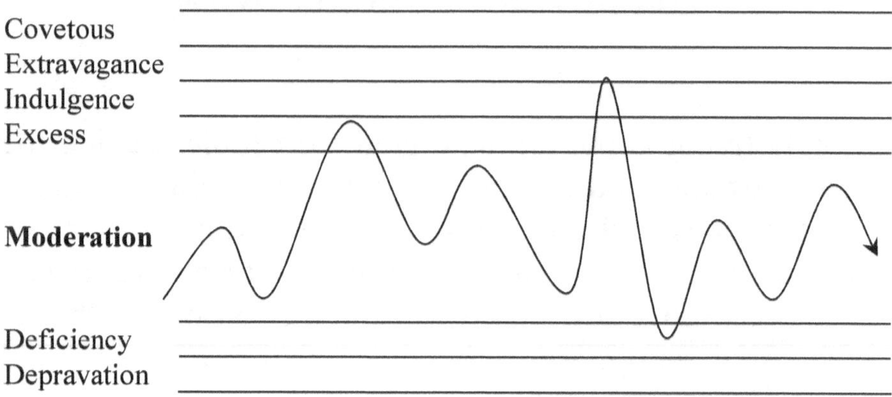

Discipline is often misunderstood, and people will often assume that discipline is only about placing restrictions on life. This is simply not true, as discipline gives you the power to act and provides you the ability to make decisions free of apprehension and uncertainty. It is vital in an age where there is a superfluous quantity of information raining down on people, leading to information exhaustion, flawed decisions, excessive consumption, and illness. Discipline is the best tool to ensure you live with a limited exposure to the information plague and the numerous pitfalls you have discovered in each part of this book.

> In choosing a way to live, a person is in effect, choosing
> a way to die.
>
> *Health-Warrior*

The foundation for this form of living takes into account all the essential human needs and is based around the following six important elements of life:

- Health and well-being

- Family and friends

- Community

- Work

- Money, consumption, and possessions

- Learning

As health and well-being is the most essential component of life (without which all the above elements of life are rendered impotent), it has been covered extensively in Part one to five of this book. Refer back to the relevant and comprehensive chapters to ensure you are empowered to make informed decisions and choices in the quest for a better health.

Family and friends

> The longer we live, and the more we think, the higher the value we learn to put on the friendship and tenderness of parents and of friends. Parents we can have but once; and he promises himself too much, who enters life with the expectation of finding many friends.
>
> *Samuel Johnson, 1766*

People adopt relationships with just about anything and everything, from objects, foods, weather, to transportation, pets, and of course other people. This can be viewed as a dilution of a person's ability to nurture meaningful and compassionate relationships with family, friends, and connections with their immediate community.

The most important relationship for a person should be the interaction with their family, where one should experience a fulfilling and positive bond with congruence in values such as love, honesty, integrity, kindness, courtesy, courage, gratitude, and patience.

The journey of life though, due to the many internal and external factors that influence and affect people, has a tendency to disrupt and dislocate these most precious relationships. In these circumstances, it would be futile to assume all family relationships were surrounded by the sweet smell of lavender and roses, and therefore, it is sometimes the case where a person has to limit their exposure to such negative relationships in order to protect their own health. However, even in these cases for your own continued emotional and physical well-being, it is important to seek peace with these family members and avoid the detrimental effects of harbouring negative feelings or emotions.

The foundations for family bonds should be laid down with the practising of daily rituals such as mealtimes (with breakfast being the most important), the way you meet and greet, evening pastimes, and sleep times. Opportunities like these nurture the sense of belonging to the family unit creating a trusting and secure environment; and it is by no means necessary to use these moments as times for communication, as it is sometimes more important to seek silence and peace than the unnecessary and trivial airspace-filling conversations. Just being in the same place at the same time is usually enough to add value to the family emotional and mental health bank. Investments of your time in the family unit will continue to show growth and maturity, promoting a positive atmosphere for communication and an acute awareness and sensitivity of the emotions and feelings of each member. All family members should seek to contribute to the success (not measured in financial terms but health and well-being ones) of the family unit, as well as friends and their immediate community.

> They seem to take away the sun from the world who withdraw friendship from life; for we have received nothing better from the immortal Gods, nothing more delightful.
>
> *Cicero*

Friends, you should be able to count on one hand; you have the power to choose who your friends are, and a wise choice will be like an addition to a loving family unit. True friendships are life-long commitments and not passing phases in a lifetime.

People you experience contact with, on the other hand, may seem just as important (at that moment in time), but they should not be seen as the complete 'friend' package. The more of these contacts you seek to maintain and nurture the increased risks of emotional fatigue and damage. In contrast, the smaller the circle of contacts the greater the opportunities for focused quality time and a more fulfilling experience.

Community

Your continued health and well-being has much to do with your immediate environment and community. It is imperative to be a proactive piece of it and contribute to its socioeconomic functioning and survival. The relationships you have with your immediate community should be one of support and cooperation, with positive experiences adding strength to values such as trust and loyalty; as with having too many contacts, you will see detrimental effects if you try to maintain excessive links within your immediate community. Fostering good relations with your neighbours can be gratifying and adds extra zest to the community spirit. However, the breaking of communication or negative relations with your neighbours can see adverse effects on your health such as increased stress levels, anxiety, and anger. There is a Mediterranean proverb which states that one bad neighbour in a street can lead to the damage of seven streets in that vicinity.

Decades ago, before the mass exodus to the cities, and the exaggerated need to house those people, one house would hold one family. In recent times, the high property prices coupled with the excess demand for accommodation has meant that, that same house has been split into numerous smaller apartments; or even just demolished for the sake of a high rise apartment building of multiple dwellings. It is very difficult to find peace of mind or body in a card stack of human beings all trying to extract their own meaning from life.

Ideally, there should be a one house per family unit quota, with the house having an adequate garden and spacing between each building. Given the choice between living in a house like this further away from the city or town (where most people work) and having to commute a further distance, or having an (inherently more expensive) apartment within the boundaries of the concrete jungle, the choice should be the house in the less populated suburbs. However, for most people, the choice is a question of convenience (living closer to places such as work, entertainment, extensive transport links, and places to eat and shop) over their health and well-being (a more peaceful environment). Is it really worth taking on the added stress and negativity of living in the city? The city propaganda machine specialises in convincing people that apartment living is a fantastic lifestyle choice. These 'fantastic' living choices are extortionately priced to hook you into city living and having to work (to repay the money borrowed) for the most appreciative years of your life. The fact that these apartments are unhealthy closed spaces packed with people one on top of the other, taking you farther away from the peace and vitality of nature and your most natural surroundings, is of little concern to anyone.

Work

> What use of health or of life if not to do some work
> therewith?
>
> *Thomas Carlyle, 1836*

Work is an essential part of human existence and commands an important place in the elements of simple living. Work performed well, will see time enthusiastically fly-by, where work is performed with resentment or in the hands of the idle, will face a torturous wait as time drags her feet. Only a person who performs work will enjoy the rich reward of rest afterwards; whereas a sedentary or an idle person will have, no idea of what rest actually is. On the other hand, work should not be excessive in duration, outside normal working times, or be unduly mentally or physically challenging, as it will be detracting from the other important parts of your life such as the time available to nurture your health, well-being, family, friends, and community.

A moderate and balanced outlook toward work should ideally see every able person work no more than thirty hours per week, while contributing to the social and economic needs of their family, be in close proximity to friends, and live within walking distance to work, in smaller neighbourhoods away from the city or towns in single-family buildings. As finding work for everybody to fit within these criteria is very difficult, within current modes of thinking, one has to try to compromise on one factor or other. One factor may have to be the choice you make in where to live in proximity to your place of work, as most forms of employment are congregated in the centres of towns or cities. The greater the distance you have between yourself and the city or town, the healthier the available living options and the lower the costs of living (housing being the single biggest cost). Therefore, a compromise may be working less hours, which means that even if you have to commute longer distances to your place of work, you will need to do it less often, making it cost efficient and more beneficial to you, and the environment. Your aims therefore, should be to create a situation of simple living, which accommodates no more than three and a half days (or thirty hours) of meaningful work providing an income to satisfy needs and comforts.

Meaningful work is something, which should provide a sense of accomplishment and a little perspiration. It is too much to ask for, if you also want it to be something that is fulfilling, satisfying, and one that adds value to your life, as those kinds of jobs are as scarce as the winning lottery ticket. It would be better for a person to work less and concentrate their efforts on contributing something back into their immediate surroundings, which could be by working in their own community or directly or indirectly donating their knowledge, contacts, support, and time. For instance, mentoring or coaching children and young adults is a great way to give something back into your place of work or immediate community. It is not all about money.

Money, consumption, and possessions

> There is no dignity quite so impressive, and no independence quite so important, as living within your means
>
> *Calvin Coolidge*

Money is not good, bad or evil, it has no power itself, only the perceived power, which people attach to it. Most times, any money you possess is money you have expended work for, and should be viewed and used accordingly. Before you can put money in its rightful place (behind health and well-being, family and friends, community, and work) in the elements of life, you need to identify and analyse your essential lifestyle needs. Look first for the necessities of life, then build up to a lifestyle, which is comfortable and not excessive or unnecessarily luxurious. This is about instilling a spending plan, as oppose to a saving one, noting that if you are not generous or have a distinct dislike for spending money you have earned, you will do yourself a great disservice as the word 'miser' originates from the word, miserable.

Do you really need all the things you say you do? Finding out your true needs is a liberating and freeing experience, and one, which will release both mental and physical energy, back into your life; as knowing your true needs will reduce or stop the effect and influence of the constant barrage of 'you need me; you deserve me; you are not living without me;' temptations of a consumerism-laced world. Concentrating on your true needs will also provide you with a greater spending power, which is the ability to extract value from all your purchases, taking into consideration the factors such as cost, durability, and quality.

Are you currently living within your means? It is a good idea to keep a track of your spending and their purposes, to identify the areas where your money goes to, and subtract it from your sources of income. The idea is not to amass as much money as you can, as this is a negative and debilitating concept. The simple living mission is to reduce your expenses and therefore, require less income to sustain a comfortable lifestyle. Basically, simple living implies that any item in your life, which does not attract an income, is an expense such as living accommodation or possessions; even if you are repaying a mortgage and car loan, for as long as you are using them, their total market value can be considered expenses. Buying increasingly bigger houses and excessively filling them with expensive furniture and appliances or purchasing cars of higher value is just increasing your expenses and adding a greater burden on your ability to produce a positive Balance of living.

Income (after tax)	Accommodation
Property rented out	Car
Shares; Bonds	House bills
Investments	Furniture, art, etc
Cash account (paying interest)	Loans & credit cards
	Insurance
Business (profitable)	Fees & charges
Pension	Sustenance
Etc.	Etc.

Income   -   **Expenses**   =   **Balance of living**

There should be no stigma attached to renting accommodation, as on most occasions it offers more favourable benefits than the loaning of money to purchase land or a house. A mortgaged house purchase is an unnecessary and speculative investment, which only continues to artificially inflate the property market and add a silver lining to the pockets of financial institutions, and the property associated parasitic businesses such as solicitors, property agents, and the insurance and assurance industries. With this in mind, you should only purchase products or services, be they a house, car, or the clothes on your back, if you have the money to pay for it outright. Not having access to these types of funds should not be a signal to be a source of revenue to others, and become attached to the vicious circle of borrowing to live. In parts of London where I lived they would refer to the action of borrowing to live, as 'buying on the never never', which implied that repaying the money for their purchases would last, what felt like an eternity before they were eventually repaid.

How much money is enough? If you have an extravagant or excessive lifestyle, then the chances are you will never quite have enough. Nevertheless, for most, having enough money is simply a positive figure in your Balance of life, for instance, where your income is greater than your expenses. How much money do you need to enjoy a loving relationship, be paid for work you enjoy, be physically active, go for a walk in the park, do some gardening, listen to music, dance, learn, be charitable, eat breakfast, drink water on a hot day, or swallow a mouthful of fresh mountainous air? The answer is not much, so the pursuit of such activities should be viewed as the richest sources of simple living, and a substantial return on your time and money investments, and actively sought and multiplied.

The investing of your money is much talked about and its every aspect exaggerated. It is always wise to note that for every winner in the speculation [read gambling] of financial markets, there is a loser, where companies can cushion heavy losses on most occasions, but the individual seldom recovers. If you truly want to live life free of preventable worry and the daily chore of tracking your financial highs and lows (not to mention the excessive charges, fees, and guesswork parading as advice), then you should stick to the lowest risk and safest financial products. You should look for a total return on your investments of around 4% (net of tax, fees, and the rate of inflation). No matter what age you are, or at what stage of life you happen to be, a return of 4% will (with regular deposits and the magic of compound interest), give you the growth required to live out the rest of your days with an adequate cash supply. As long as you do not draw on more than 2 to 3% yearly from your main capital lump sum.

Simple living reduces the need for excessive consumption or surplus possessions; where excessive is anything more than fulfilling of a need or being beyond useful. There should be no room for relationship development in anything consumed or purchased, and anything past its useful service date should be recycled (all possessions should be recyclable in some for or other). Avoiding being absorbed and immersed in the pursuit and purchase of possessions, and a person will recognise the fact there is little connection between the purchases and their life fulfilment. They will observe that the unwarranted accumulation of possessions will only corrupt their search for a healthier and happier life, and should ultimately become aware of the increasing need to overcome such habits, which only produce temporary gratification of the senses and increasing profits for others.

A clutter-free and simple living environment is essential for optimum health and well-being, therefore, any reduction in your consumption or accumulation of possessions should be seen as wise investment in your Balance of living.

Learning

Learning is ever young, even in old age.

Aeschylus, c.490BC

The anchor element in the pursuit of a simple life is learning. It is the wheels on which all the other elements move, and a guiding star with which to navigate successfully away from the obstacles, dangers, and enticements of a modern life, and toward the achievement, contentment, and peace of mind. As with all the elements of life, even learning has, its roots set firmly in moderation and balance. Sometimes the most important lessons, come from not only knowing what to do with what you have learned, but also knowing what not to do with it, where inaction is just as crucial as, and often more crucial than, action.

These recent decades have been dubbed the 'Information Age', where knowledge and information is seen as a valuable commodity. However, the greatest myth and tragedy of this age, is that there is a vast plethora of biased, incorrect, and useless items of information, which are thrown at people from every angle, making it virtually impossible for any person to decipher any useful morsels of knowledge. Learning is much more than the absorption and recall ability of facts or theories, or a how-to life instruction manual. People spending the majority of their time ingesting fashionable information and knowledge streams, are just hampering the real aim of learning, the ability to think.

Enjoying a playful and questioning childhood, being a contrarian and a frugal scholar in your teens, and a student of life from your twenty years onwards should see that you are graced with the wisdom needed for a sophisticated and simple way of learning and living.

...schools fit us for the university rather than for the world.

John Locke

Children, before they are tainted by schooling (and parents), are curious, excited by and inspired by their ability to learn. If children where left to their own means and instincts, they would learn naturally and pursue a way of living which is ideal for them. However, schooling has the tendency to suffocate and extinguish this natural curiosity and excitement. Instead of using their desire to learn, to supply them with the tools on how to think, they are plied with a structured and monotonous one-size-fits-all education ('instruction'). How relevant is that fact that one child knows a little more than another does? Unfortunately, for countless years now, it has been seen as the difference between success and failure; with where you went to school, college, or university a badge of honour, and maybe worse still, admired as such. Schooling forfeits much of the growth years of living when it stubbornly follows a path of instruction, which is of little relevance and use on the day of graduation.

How much of what you learned during your school years do you use in your everyday life? For most people, learning only really starts the day after leaving the education system. How many people do you know who manage to graduate from the school of life? Sadly, until then it is a fact that the regurgitation of memorised facts, concepts, and theories is worth more than true learning, where true learning is the training of the mind to think, and one, which will grow from the joy, curiosity, and discipline of living and the cultivation of the power of observation.

True learning is the preparation for living and one, which is better learned through enjoyment than it is ever learned by forced lessons of misfortune. To make any strides forward in learning, you would do a lot worse than to heed the following words of Mill.

> A cultivated mind, I do not mean that of a philosopher, but any mind to which the fountains of knowledge have been opened, and which has been taught in any tolerable degree to exercise its faculties—will find sources of inexhaustible interest in all that surrounds it; in the objects of nature, the achievements of art, the imaginations of poetry, the incidents of history, the ways of mankind, past and present, and their prospects in the future. It is possible, indeed, to become indifferent to all this, and that too without having exhausted a thousandth part of it; but only when one has had from the beginning no moral or human interest in these things, and has sought in them only the gratification of curiosity.
>
> *John S. Mill*

The Health-Warrior constitution

Principles are personal; and ones that you have developed through childhood and life experience, creating an unwritten list of behaviour criteria, which you carry throughout life. It is your day-to-day behaviour, which will determine and define your guiding principles. However, more often than not, these principles are a checklist for the way a person believes other people should behave toward them, rather than being the guide for their behaviour toward others. Make a daily difference and lead by example, here are the leading lights for the Health-Warrior in you:

- Lead the fight against the forces of ill health and disease
- Display an unerring commitment to live life with honesty and integrity
- Nurture loving and trusting relationships
- Show courtesy, compassion, and kindness to others
- Enjoy nature at every available moment and minimise the personal and collective environmental footprint left on the Earth
- Take responsibility for every word, thought, and action
- Utilise the power of positivity
- Continually seek to develop discipline and balance to realise optimum vitality
- Invest wisely in spiritual, emotional, physical and mental health
- Draw deep from the well of wisdom, and seek the counsel of others such as the contrarian, devil's advocate, or cynic, to make informed decisions and choices
- Live simply and modestly with sustainable consumption
- Adopt a modest financial budget and minimise risks taken with money
- Seek to reduce working commitment to less than thirty hours per week
- Reduce the reliance on money, and material goods or amusement experiences
- Contribute and cooperate to the success of the family, friends, and immediate community
- Promote positive habits with affirmation, recognition, incentive, and reward

If you have the heart of a Health-Warrior, you have health, if you have health, you have hope, and if you have hope, you have everything.

Bibliography and Resources

Health-Warrior website: health-warrior.co.uk

Email: info@health-warrior.co.uk

Part one – Air power

Wanda Phipatanakul, Allergic Rhinoconjunctivitis: Epidemiology. Immunol Allergy Clin North Am. 2005 May ; 25(2): 263–vi.

Isaac N. Luginaah, et al. Association of Ambient Air Pollution with Respiratory Hospitalization in a Government-Designated "Area of Concern": The Case of Windsor, Ontario. Environ Health Perspect 113:290–296 (2005).

Beggs PJ, Bambrick HJ. Is the Global Rise of Asthma an Early Impact of Anthropogenic Climate Change? Environ Health Perspect 113:915–919 (2005).

Roitman JL, Herridge M et al. ACSM's resource manual for Guidelines for exercise testing and prescription. American College of Sports Medicine – 4th ed. Lippincott Williams & Wilkins, Philadelphia, 2001.

Berger AJ. Control of breathing. In Murray JF, Nadel JA, eds. Textbook of Respiratory Medicine, vol 1. 2nd ed. Philadelphia, Saunders, 1994:199-218.

McArdale WD, Katch FI, Katch VL. Exercise Physiology: Energy, Nutrition, and Human Performance. 5th ed. Lippincott Williams & Wilkins, Philadelphia, 2001.

Clifford PS, et al. Arterial blood pressure response to rowing. Med Sci Sports Exerc 1994;26:715

Gaffney FA, et al. Cardiovascular and metabolic responses to static contraction in man. Acta Physiol Scand 1990;138:249.

Lassen A, et al. Cardiovascular responses to static contractions in man with topical nerve blockade. J Physiol (Lond) 1989;409:333

MacDougall D, et al. Arterial blood pressure response to resistance exercise. J Appl Physiol 1985;58:785

Smith MA, et al. Assessment of beat to beat changes in cardiac output during the Valsalva manoeuvre using bioimpedence cardiology. Clin Sci 1987;72:423

Ten Harkel ADJ, et al. Assessment of cardiovascular reflexes: influence of posture and period of preceding rest. J Appl Physiol 1990;68:147

Black O, Bailey S. The Mind Gym. Time Warner Books, London, 2005

Bernardi L, et al. Effect of breathing rate on oxygen saturation and exercise performance on chronic heart failure. The Lancet 1998;351:9112:1308-1311

Holford P, Cass H. Natural Highs. Piatkus, London, 2001

Vogel HC. The Nature Doctor. Mainstream Publishing, Edinburgh, 1990.

Fried R. The Breath Connection. Plenum Press, New York, 1990

Fried R, Grimaldi J. The Psychology and Physiology of Breathing in Behavioural Medicine, Clinical Psychology, and Psychiatry. Plenum Press, New York, 1993

Cohen KS. The Way of Qigong; The art and science of Chinese energy healing. Bantam Books, London, 1997

Taqi-ud-Din Al-Hilai M, Khan MM. The Noble Qur'an: Transliteration in Roman Script with Arabic text and English. Darusssalam, Riyadh, 1996

The Bible. King James Version, Old Testament, Genesis, 2:7

Arnold E. The Bhagavad-Gita. (Translated from the Sanskrit Text), Truslove, Hanson & Comba, New York, 1900

Yogananda P, Autobiography of a YOGI. Encinitis, California, 1945

Eastman CA. The Soul Of The Indian: An Interpretation by Charles Alexander Eastman

Eastman CA. Indian Boyhood: An Interpretation by Charles Alexander Eastman

Besant A. An Introduction to Yoga. Lectures delivered at 32nd Anniversary of the Theosophical Society held at Benares, on Dec. 27th, 28th, 29th, and 30th, 1907.

Brown C. The Yoga Bible: The definitive guide to yoga postures. Godsfield Press, Alresford, 2003.

Parker KL. The Euahlayi Tribe--A Study of Aboriginal Life in Australia

Nukariyan K. The Religion of the Samurai: A Study of Zen Philosophy and Discipline in China and Japan. Tokyo, 1913

Shaykh Hakim Moinuddin Chishti. The Book of Sufi Healing. Inner Traditions, Rochester, Vermont, 1991

Dahl R. Heavy Traffic Ahead: Car Culture Accelerates. Environ Health Perspect. 2005 April; 113(4): A238–A245

Gilliland et al. Air Pollution Exposure Assessment for Epidemiologic Studies of Pregnant Women and Children: Lessons Learned from the Centers for Children's Environmental Health and Disease Prevention Research. Environ Health Perspect 113:1447–1454 (2005). doi:10.1289/ehp.7673

Künzli et al. Ambient Air Pollution and Atherosclerosis in Los Angeles. Environ Health Perspect; 113(2): 201–206. February 2005. doi: 10.1289/ehp.7523

Riediker et al. Cardiovascular effects in patrol officers are associated with fine particulate matter from brake wear and engine emissions. Part Fibre Toxicol. 2004; 1: 2. doi: 10.1186/1743-8977-1-2.

Kessler R. Death by Particles: The Link between Air Pollution and Fatal Coronary Heart Disease in Women. Environ Health Perspect. 2005 December; 113(12): A836–A837

Schikowski T et al. Long-term air pollution exposure and living close to busy roads are associated with COPD in women. Respiratory Research 2005, 6:152 doi:10.1186/1465-9921-6-152

Lie Hong Chen et al. The Association between Fatal Coronary Heart Disease and Ambient Particulate Air Pollution: Are Females at Greater Risk? Environ Health Perspect 113:1723–1729 (2005). doi:10.1289/ehp.8190

Spivey A. On Closer Inspection: Learning to look at the Whole Home Environment. Environmental Health Perspectives, Volume 113, Number 5, May 2005: A 321-3 University of California at Berkeley Wellness Letter 12(5) February 1996

Sachs DPL. Cigarette smoking: Health effects and cessation strategies. Clin Geriatr Med 2:337-362, 1986

Schuman LM. The benefits of cessation of smoking. Chest 59:421-427, 1971

Beggs PJ. Is the Global Rise of Asthma an Early Impact of Anthropogenic Climate Change? Environ Health Perspect 113:915–919 (2005). doi:10.1289/ehp.7724

Britton et al. British Lung Foundation, Lung Report III – Casting a shadow over the nation's health. ISBN 0 9527472 0 0. 2005

Hershovitz J. Environmental Health Perspectives Vol. 113 No. 5 May 2005

Bhatia R, Lopipero P, Smith AH. 1998. Diesel exhaust and lung cancer. Epidemiology 9(1):84–91.

Lipsett M, Campleman S. 1999. Occupational exposure to diesel exhaust and lung cancer: a meta-analysis. Am J Public Health 89(7):1009–1017.

Garshick E et al. Lung Cancer in Railroad Workers Exposed to Diesel Exhaust. Environ Health Perspect 112:1539–1543 (2004). doi:10.1289/ehp.7195

Donaldson K et al. Combustion-derived nanoparticles: A review of their toxicology following inhalation exposure. Particle and Fibre Toxicology 2005, 2:10 doi:10.1186/1743-8977-2-10. This article is available from: www.particleandfibretoxicology.com/content/2/1/10

Sheridan M. Deadly dust of gem trade kills Chinese. The Sunday Times, March 26, 2006; 1.27

Hoet PHM et al. Nanoparticles – known and unknown health risks. Journal of Nanobiotechnology 2004, 2:12 doi:10.1186/1477-3155-2-12. This article is available from: www.jnanobiotechnology.com/content/2/1/12

Wilhelm M et al. Local Variations in CO and Particulate Air Pollution and Adverse Birth Outcomes in Los Angeles County, California, USA. Environ Health Perspect 113:1212–1221 (2005) doi:10.1289/ehp.7751

Bernardi L et al. Effect of breathing rate on oxygen on saturation and exercise performance in chronic heart failure. The Lancet, 351, 9112, 1308-1311 (1998)

Watts J. Beijing to ban drivers for blue sky Olympics. Guardian Unlimited (Friday April 7, 2006) Reuters (Berlin). EU to take Germany to court over tobacco ads: report (Wed Apr 12, 2006 7:32am ET)

Resources

www.airquality.co.uk	UK Air Quality
www.appliedozone.com	Ozone air / water purifier
www.who.int	World Health Organisation
www.defra.gov.uk/	UK Government Environment air quality statistics
www.epa.gov/iaq	Division of the National Safety Council, Washington, DC
www.lunguk.org	British Lung Foundation
www.battelle.org	Organisation identifying future trends

Part two – Elixir of life

Holford P, Cass H. Natural Highs. Piatkus, London, 2001

McArdale WD, Katch FI, Katch VL. Exercise Physiology: Energy, Nutrition, and Human Performance. 5th ed. Lippincott Williams & Wilkins, Philadelphia, 2001.

Cohen KS. The Way of Qigong; The art and science of Chinese energy healing. Bantam Books, London, 1997

Nukariyan K. The Religion of the Samurai: A Study of Zen Philosophy and Discipline in China and Japan. Tokyo, 1913.

Hippocrates. On Airs, Waters, and Places. Translated by Francis Adams. Provided by The Internet Classics Archive, Online - http://classics.mit.edu//Hippocrates/airwatpl.html

Swaka MN, et al. Influence of body water and blood volume on the thermoregulatio and exercise performance in the heat. Exerc Sport Sci Rev, 27:167; 1999.

Caldwell JE, et al. Diuretic therapy, physical performance, and neuromuscular function. Phys Sports Med; 12:73; 1984.

Shirreffs SM, Maughan RJ. Restoration of fluid balance after exercise. Exer Spor Sci Rev; 1:27; 2000

Evans EP. Animal Symbolism In Ecclesiastical Architecture. W. Heinemann, London. 1896

Wallace Budge EA. Legends of the Gods.

Lathe R. Autism, Brain and Environment. Jessica Kingsley, London. 2006.

BBC World Service. Earth Report. Screened 06.30 GMT. 12th February 2006.

World Health Organisation. Water sanitation and health guidelines; www.who.int/water_sanitation_health/dwq/guidelines/en/

World Health Organisation. Arsenic in drinking water. Fact sheet N°210,Revised May 2001

Rose JB. et al, Climate Variability and Change in the United States: Potential Impacts on Waterand Foodborne Diseases Caused by Microbiologic Agents. Environ Health Perspect 109(suppl 2):211–221 2001.

Bottled water bacteria. Arch Fam Med 2000; 9:246-250

Altmann P, et al. Disturbance of cerebral function in people exposed to drinking water contaminated with aluminium sulphate: retrospective study of the Camelford water incident. BMJ 1999;319:807–11

Lack T. Water and health in Europe: an overview. BMJ ;318:1678–82; 1999

Walker A. Drinking water - doubts about quality. Br Med J. 304: 175; 1992

Allen HE, Halley-Henderson MA, Hass CN. Chemical composition of bottled mineral water. Arch Environ Hlth. 44: 102; 1989

National Research Council, National Academy of Sciences: Toxicity Testing: Strategies to Determine Needs and Priorities. National Academy Press, 1984

LaDou J: The clinical significance of water pollution. Medical Staff Conference. West J Med 1988 Feb; 148:192-196. 1988.

Hunter PR, Burge SH. The bacteriological quality of bottled natural mineral waters. Epidemiol Infect; 99: 43; 1987.

Ministry of Agriculture, Fisheries and Food. The Natural Mineral Water Regulations. Statutory Instruments No 71 . London: HMSO, 1985.

United Nations World Water Development Report. 2005

Metabolites Of Pharmaceuticals Identified In Wastewater. Research Center, University of Buffalo, State University of New York. March 2006.

Ebbeling C, et al. Soft drinks gain weight. Pediatircs. USA. March 2006.

Savona N. The Kitchen Shrink: Foods and recipes for a healthy mind. Duncan Baird Publishers. London. 2003

Resources

www.epa.gov/OW/you/chap3.html	United States
www.americanwater.com/49ways.htm	United States
www.water.org.uk/	United Kingdom
www.defra.gov.uk/environment/water/conserve/save.htm	United Kingdom
www.waterconserve.info/	Australia

Part three – Nourishment

Levine AS et al. Effect of breakfast cereals on short-term food intake. Am J Clin Nutr. 1989 Dec;50(6):1303-7

Kirby RW, et al. Oat bran intake selectively lowers serum low density lipoprotein cholesterol concentrations of hyper-cholesterolemic men. Am J Clin Nutr 1981; 34:824

Willett W, et al. Glycemic index, glycemic load, and risk of type 2 diabetes. Am J Clin Nutr. 2002;76(1):274S-280S.

Liu S, et al. Dietary glycemic load and atherothrombotic risk. Curr Atheroscler Rep. 2002;4(6):454-461.

Foster-Powell K, et al. International table of glycemic index and glycemic load values: 2002. Am J Clin Nutr. 2002;76(1):5-56.

Willett W, et al. Glycemic index, glycemic load, and risk of type 2 diabetes. Am J Clin Nutr. 2002;76(1):274S-280S. (PubMed)

Salmeron J,et al. Dietary fiber, glycemic load, and risk of non-insulin-dependent diabetes mellitus in women. JAMA. 1997;277(6):472-477.

Wolever T, et al. Prediction of glucose and insulin responses of normal subjects after consuming mixed meals varying in energy, protein, fat, carbohydrate and glycemic index.. J Nutr 1996, 126:2807-2812.

Galani J, et al. Acute effect of meal glycemic index and glycemic load on blood glucose and insulin responses in humans. Nutrition Journal 2006, 5:22 doi:10.1186/1475-2891-5-22. Available at: www.nutritionj.com/content/5/1/22

Sheard N, et al. Dietary carbohydrate (amount and type) in the prevention and management of diabetes: a statement by the American Diabetes Association. Diabetes Care 2004, 27:2266-2271.

Brand-Miller J, et al. Low-Glycemic Index Diets in the Management of Diabetes: A meta-analysis of randomized controlled trials. Diabetes Care. 2003;26(8):2261-2267.

Ford ES, et al. Glycemic index and serum high-density lipoprotein cholesterol concentration among us adults. Arch Intern Med. 2001;161(4):572-576.

Liu S, et al. Dietary glycemic load assessed by food-frequency questionnaire in relation to plasma high-density-lipoprotein cholesterol and fasting plasma triacylglycerols in postmenopausal women. Am J Clin Nutr. 2001;73(3):560-566.

Ludwig DS. Dietary glycemic index and the regulation of body weight. Lipids. 2003;38(2):117-121.

Ebbeling CB, et al. A reduced-glycemic load diet in the treatment of adolescent obesity. Arch Pediatr Adolesc Med 2003;157:773–9. [PubMed: 12912783]

Silvera SA, et al. Dietary carbohydrates and breast cancer risk: a prospective study of the roles of overall glycemic index and glycemic load. Int J Cancer. 2005;114(4):653-658.

Higginbotham S, et al. Dietary glycemic load and breast cancer risk in the Women's Health Study. Cancer Epidemiol Biomarkers Prev. 2004;13(1):65-70.

Michaud DS, et al. Dietary sugar, glycemic load, and pancreatic cancer risk in a prospective study. J Natl Cancer Inst. 2002;94(17):1293-1300.

Higginbotham S, et al. Dietary glycemic load and risk of colorectal cancer in the Women's Health Study. J Natl Cancer Inst. 2004;96(3):229-233.

Horne M. Health food? Try a dog's dinner. The Sunday Times, March 26, 2006. News 1, p.3

Hu FB, et al. Dietary fat intake and the risk of coronary heart disease in women. New England J Med 1997;337:1491.

Arita M,et al. Stereochemical assignment, anti-inflammatory properties, and receptor for the omega-3 lipid mediator resolvin E1. J Exp Med. 2005 Mar 7;201(5):713-22.

Andreassi, M,et al. Efficacy of Gamma Linolenic Acid in the treatment of patients with atopic dermatitis. Journal of International Medical Research. 1997 25:286.

Brush, MG,et al.. Abnormal essential fatty acid levels in plasma of women with premenstrual syndrome. Amer. Journal Obstet. Gynecol. 1984 150:363-356.

Pullman-Mooar S., et al. Alteration of the cellular fatty acid profile and the production of eicosanoids in human monocytes by gamma-linolenic acid. Arthritis and Rheumatism. 1990 33:1526-33.

Tate, G., et al. Suppression of acute and chronic inflammation by dietary gamma linolenic acid. J. Rheumatol. 1989 16:729.

Ziboh, V.A. 1998. Lipoxygenation of Gamma Linolenic Acid by skin epidermis: Modulation of epidermal inflammatory/hyperproliferative processes. Proceedings of the Annual Meeting of the American Oil Chemists' Society.1998 pp. 25.

Zurier, RB., et al. Gamma-linolenic acid, inflammation, immune responses and Rheumatoid Arthritis. In: Gamma-linolenic acid: Metabolism and its roles in nutrition and medicine. Huang Y-S and Mills, D.E., Eds., AOCS Press, Champaign, Illinois. 1996 pp. 129-136.

Melnick, B., et al. Atopic dermatitis and disturbances in essential fatty acid and prostaglandin E metabolism. J.Amer. Acad. Dermatol. 1991;25:859

Diezel W E, et al. Plant oils: Topical application and anti-inflammatory effects (croton oil test). Dermatol. Monatsschr. 1993;179:173

Nissen, H P, et al. The effects of gamma linolenic acid on skin smoothness, humidity and TEWL - A clinical study. Inform 1995;6;4:5 19

Ruano J, et al. Phenolic content of virgin olive oil improves ischemic reactive hyperemia in hypercholesterolemic patients. J Am Coll Cardiol. 2005 Nov 15;46(10):1864-8., PMID: 16286173

Aguilera CM, et al. Protective effect of monounsaturated and polyunsaturated fatty acids on the development of cardiovascular disease]. Nutr Hosp 2001 May-2001 Jun 30;16(3):78-91, PMID: 11620

Caponio F, et al. Influence of the exposure to light on extra virgin olive oil quality during storage. European Food Research and Technology, 2005 July; 221(1-2):92-98.

Garcia-Segovia P, et al. Olive oil consumption and risk of breast cancer in the Canary Islands: a population-based case-control study. Public Health Nutr 2006 Feb;9(1A):163-7., PMID: 16512965

Gill CI, et al. Potential anti-cancer effects of virgin olive oil phenols on colorectal carcinogenesis models in vitro. Int J Cancer. 2005 Oct 20;117(1):1-7., PMID: 15880398

Psaltopoulou T, et al. Olive oil, the Mediterranean diet, and arterial blood pressure: the Greek European Prospective Investigation into Cancer and Nutrition (EPIC) study. Am J Clin Nutr. 2004 Oct;80(4):1012-8., PMID: 15447913

Mozaffarian D, et al. Trans fatty acids and cardiovascular disease. N Engl J Med. 2006 Apr 13;354(15):1601-13.

Booyens J, et al. The role of unnatural dietary trans and cis unsaturated fatty acids in the epidemiology of coronary artery disease Med Hypotheses 1988; 25:175-182.

Mensink RPM, et al. Effect of dietary trans fatty acids on high-density and low-density lipoprotein cholesterol levels in healthy subjects. N Engl J Med 1990; 323:439-45.

Willett WC, et al. Trans fatty acids: Are the effects only marginal? Am J Public Health 1994; 84:722-724.

Martin MJ, et al. Serum cholestero, blood pressure, and mortality: implications from a coort of 361,663 men. Lancet 1986;2:933.

Lipid Research Clinic Program: The lipid clinics coronary primary prevention trial results. I. The relationship of the reduction in incidence of coronary heart diseas to cholesterol lowering. JAMA 1984;251:351.

Lipid Research Clinic Program: The lipid clinics coronary primary prevention trial results. II. The relationship of the reduction in incidence of coronary heart disease to cholesterol lowering. JAMA 1984;251:365.

Kerstetter JE, et al. Dietary protein, calcium metabolism, and skeletal homeostasis revisited. Am J Clin Nutr. 2003 Sep;78(3 Suppl):584S-592S

Young VR, et al. Plant proteins in relation to human protein and amino acid nutrition. Am J Clin Nutr 1994;59 (supplement):1203S–12S.

David G. The pattern of world protein consumption Geoforum: Volume 26, Issue 1 , February 1995, Pages 1-17. doi:10.1016/0016-7185(94)00020-8.

Food & Agriculture Organization/World Health Organization/United Nations University (1985). Energy & protein requirements. WHO Technical Report Series 724. Geneva: WHO.

Lappé, F.M. (1976). Diet for a Small Planet. New York: Ballantine Books.

Millward, D.J., et al (1992). Amino acid scoring in health and disease. In: Protein-Energy Interactions - Proceedings of a workshop held by the International Dietary Energy Consultancy Group. Switzerland: IDECG.

Heaney R. Protein intake and the calcium economy. J Am Diet Assoc 1993;93:1259–60 [review].

Abelow BJ, et al. Cross-cultural association between dietary animal protein and hip fracture: a hypothesis. Calcif Tiss Int 1992;50:14–8.

Hoeksma M, et al. The intake of total protein, natural protein and protein substitute and growth of height and head circumference in Dutch infants with phenylketonuria. Journal of Inherited Metabolic Disease. Biomedical and Life Sciences , Issue Volume 28, Number 6 / December, 2005 .DOI 10.1007/s10545-005-0122-x .Pages 845-854.

Yusuf S, et al. Vitamin E supplementation and cardiovascular events in high-risk patients. The Heart Outcomes Prevention Evaluation Study Investigators. N Engl J Med 2000; 342:154-60.

Kris-Etherton PM, et al. American Heart Association science advisory: antioxidant vitamin supplements and cardiovascular disease. Circulation 2004; 110:637-641

Beecher C. Cancer preventive properties of varieties of Brassica oleracea: a review. Am J Clin Nutr 1994;59(Suppl):1166S-70S 1994

Dinkova-Kostova AT, et al. Protection against UV-light-induced skin carcinogenesis in SKH-1 high-risk mice by sulforaphane-containing broccoli sprout extracts. Cancer Lett. 2005 Nov 2; [Epub ahead of print], PMID: 16271437

Huxley RR, et al. The relation between dietary flavonol intake and coronary heart disease mortality: a meta-analysis of prospective cohort studies,. European Journal of Clinical Nutrition (2003) 57, 904-908.

Fahey JW, et al. Sulforaphane inhibits extracellular, intracellular, and antibiotic-resistant strains of Helicobacter pylori and prevents benzopyrene-induced stomach tumors. Proc Natl Acad Sci USA 2002 May 28;99(11):7610-5 2002

Gaziano JM, et al. A prospective study of consumption of carotenoids in fruits and vegetables and decreased cardiovascular mortality in the elderly. Ann. Epidemiol. 1995; 5:255-260.

Michaud DS, et al. Intake of specific carotenoids and risk of lung cancer in 2 prospective US cohorts. Am J Clin Nutr(2000)Oct;72(4):990-7.

Harris RA, et al. A case-controlled study of dietary carotene in men with lung cancer. Nutrition and Cancer(1991)15:63-68

Kobaek-Larsen M, et al. Inhibitory Effects of Feeding with Carrots or (-)-Falcarinol on Development of Azoxymethane-Induced Preneoplastic Lesions in the Rat Colon. J Agric Food Chem. 2005 Mar 9;53(5):1823-1827.

Feskanich D, et al. Prospective study of fruit and vegetable consumption and risk of lung cancer among men and women. J Natl Cancer Inst 2000, 92:1812-1823.

Le Marchand L, et al. Intake of flavonoids and lung cancer. J Natl Canc Inst 2000, 92:154-160.

Sun J, et al. Antioxidant and anti proliferative activities of common fruits. J Agric Food Chem 2002, 50:7449-7454.

Eberhardt M, et al. Antioxidant activity of fresh apples. Nature 2000, 405:903-904.

Aprikian O, et al. Apple pectin and a polyphenols rich apple concentrate are more effective together than separately on cecal fermentations and plasma lipids in rats. J Nutr 2003, 133:1860-1865.

Sesso H, et al. Flavonoid intake and risk of cardiovascular disease in women..Am J Clin Nutr 2003, 77:1400-1408.

Knekt P, et al. Flavonoid intake and risk of chronic diseases. Am J Clin Nutr 2002, 76:560-568.

Tabak C, et al. Chronic obstructive pulmonary disease and intake of catechins, flavonols, and flavones. Am J Respir Crit Care Med 2001, 164:61-64.

de Oliviera M, et al. Weight loss associated with a daily intake of three apples or three pears among overweight women. Nutr 2003, 19:253-256.

Boyer J. et al. Apple phytochemicals and their health benefits. Department of Food Science and Institute of Comparative and Environmental Toxicology, Nutrition Journal 2004, 3:5 doi:10.1186/1475-2891-3-5.

Andreadou I, et al. The olive constituent oleuropein exhibits anti-ischemic, antioxidative, and hypolipidemic effects in anesthetized rabbits. J Nutr. 2006 Aug;136(8):2213-9.

Hamdi HK, et al. Oleuropein, a non-toxic olive iridoid, is an anti-tumor agent and cytoskeleton disruptor. Biochem Biophys Res Commun. 2005 Sep 2;334(3):769-78

Juan ME, et al. Olive Fruit Extracts Inhibit Proliferation and Induce Apoptosis in HT-29 Human Colon Cancer Cells. J Nutr. 2006 Oct;136(10):2553-7.

O'Brien NM, et al. Modulatory effects of resveratrol, citroflavan-3-ol, and plant-derived extracts on oxidative stress in U937 cells. J Med Food. 2006 Summer;9(2):187-95.

Martinez-Dominguez E, et al. Protective effects upon experimental inflammation models of a polyphenol-supplemented virgin olive oil diet. Inflamm Res 2001; 50(2): 102-6.

Zhan S, et al. Meta-analysis of the effects of soy protein containing isoflavones on the lipid profile. Am J Clin Nutr 2005;81:397-408.

Colacurci N, et al. Effects of soy isoflavones on endothelial function in healthy postmenopausal women. Menopause 2005;12:299-307.

Lissin LW, et al. Isoflavones improve vascular reactivity in post-menopausal women with hypercholesterolemia. Vasc Med 2004;9:26-30.

He J, et al. Effect of soy bean protein on blood pressure: a randomized, controlled trial. Ann Intern Med 2005;143:1-9.

Brouwer IA, et al. Dietary alpha-linolenic acid is associated with reduced risk of fatal coronary heart disease, but increased prostate cancer risk: a meta-analysis. J Nutr 2004;134:919-922.

Zhang X, et al. Soy food consumption is associated with lower risk of coronary heart disease in Chinese women. J Nutr 2003;133:2874-2878.

Naaz A, et al. The soy isoflavone genistein decreases adipose deposition in mice. Endocrinology. Aug 2003; 144(8):3315-20.

Chen YM, et al. Soy isoflavones have a favorable effect on bone loss in Chinese postmenopausal women with lower bone mass: a double-blind, randomized, controlled trial. J Clin Endocrinol Metab. 2003 Oct;88(10):4740-7.

Kritz-Silverstein D, et al. Usual dietary isoflavone intake, bone mineral density, and bone metabolism in postmenopausal women. J Womens Health Gend Based Med 2002 Jan-Feb;11(1):69-78.

Teixeira SR, et al. Isolated soy protein consumption reduces urinary albumin excretion and improves the serum lipid profile in men with type 2 diabetes mellitus and nephropathy. J Nutr. 2004 Aug;134(8):1874-80.

Sagara M, et al. Effects of dietary intake of soy protein and isoflavones on cardiovascular disease risk factors in high risk, middle-aged men in Scotland. J Am Coll Nutr. 2004 Feb;23(1):85-91.

Guo JY, et al. Dietary soy isoflavones and estrone protect ovariectomized ERalphaKO and wild-type mice from carcinogen-induced colon cancer. J Nutr. 2004 Jan;134(1):179-82.

Wood CE, et al. Breast and uterine effects of soy isoflavones and conjugated equine estrogens in postmenopausal female monkeys. J Clin Endocrinol Metab. 2004 Jul;89(7):3462-8.

Wien MA, et al. Almonds vs complex carbohydrates in a weight reduction program. Int J Obes Relat Metab Disord. 2003 Nov;27(11):1365-72.

Chen CY, et al. Flavonoids from almond skins are bioavailable and act synergistically with vitamins C and E to enhance hamster and human LDL resistance to oxidation. J Nutr. 2005 Jun;135(6):1366-73.

Sang S, et al. Sphingolipid and other constituents from almond nuts (Prunus amygdalus Batsch). J Agric Food Chem 2002; 50:4709-4712.

Scott LW, et al. Long-term, randomonized clinical trial of two diets in the metabolic syndrome and type 2 diabetes. Diabetes Care 2003; 26(8): 2481-2.

Davis P, et al. Whole almonds and almond fractions reduce aberrant crypt foci in a rat model of colon carcinogenesis. Cancer Letters 2001; 165:27-33.

Hyson DA, et al. Almonds and almond oil have similar effects on plasma lipid and LDL oxidation in healthy men and women. J Nutr 2002; 132(4):703-7.

Fulgoni V. Almonds lower blood cholesterol and LDL-cholesterol but not HDL-cholestero or triglycerides in human subjects: results of a meta-analysis. Presented at Experimental Biology, 2002.

G.P.Lim et al. Polyunsaturated fatty acid (PUFA) intake alters levels of b-amyloid and insulin degrading enzyme in aged Alzheimer mouse model. Program No. 544.16. 2005 Abstract Viewer/Itinerary Planner. Washington, DC: Society for Neuroscience, 2005.

Almonds, daily exercise keep brain healthy. By Kathleen Fackelmann, USA TODAY Posted 11/14/2005 8:48 PM. www.usatoday.com/news/health/2005-11-14-brain-almonds-health_x.htm

Bazzano LA, et al. Dietary fiber intake and reduced risk of coronary heart disease in US men and women: the National Health and Nutrition Examination Survey I Epidemiologic Follow-up Study. Arch Intern Med. 2003 Sep 8;163(16):1897-904

Tsikitis VL, et al. Beta-glucan affects leukocyte navigation in a complex chemotactic gradient. Surgery. 2004 Aug;136(2):384-9.

Liu RH. New finding may be key to ending confusion over link between fiber, colon cancer. American Institute for Cancer Research Press Release, November 3, 2004.

Johnsen N et al. Intake of whole grains and vegetables determines the plasma enterolactone concentration of Danish women. J Nutr. 2004 Oct;134(10):2691-7.

Your Guide To Lowering Your Blood Pressure With DASH. U.S. Department of Health and Human Services, National Institutes of Health, National Heart, Lung, and Blood Institute; NIH Publication No. 06-4082. Originally Printed 1998.Revised April 2006

Bendich A et al. Potential health economic benefits of vitamin supplementation. West J Med. 1997 May; 166(5): 306–312.

Megarry, Tim (1995) Society in Prehistory: The Origins of Human Culture. New York: New York University Press.

Walker, Alan and Shipman, Pat (1996) The Wisdom of the Bones: In Search of Human Origins. New York: Alfred A. Knopf.

Burenhult, Goran (ed.) (1993a). The First Humans: Human Origins and History to 10,000 B.C. New York: Harper-Collins Publishers.

Eaton, S. Boyd (1992) "Humans, Lipids, and Evolution." Lipids, vol. 27, no. 10 .1992

How to Cure Obesity. The Washington Post - Washington, D.C. Nov 15, 1885

Quigley, DT. The National Malnutrition. The Lee Foundation for Nutritional Research Milwaukee, Wisconsin 1943

Bogert LJ, Nutrition and Physical Fitness, Philadelphia: Saunders, 1939:437.

Eaton SB, Shostak M, and Konner M, The Paleolithic Prescription: A program of diet & exercise and a design for living, New York: Harper & Row, 1988:39.

Cordain L. Origins and evolution of the Western diet: health implications for the 21st century1,2. Am J Clin Nutr 2005;81:341–54.

Temple NJ, Burkitt DP: Western diseases: their dietary prevention and reversibility. Totowa, NJ, Humana Press; 1994

Jonsson T et al. Agrarian diet and diseases of affluence – Do evolutionary novel dietary lectins cause leptin resistance? BMC Endocrine Disorders 2005, 5:10 doi:10.1186/1472-6823-5-10 This article is available from: www.biomedcentral.com/1472-6823/5/10

UK Heart Disease Mortality rates available at: www.heartstats.org/uploads/documents%5CCh1_Mortality_2005.pdf

British Heart Foundation. Statistics Database. www.heartstats.org

American Heart Association. Heart Disease and Stroke Statistics—2005 Update. Dallas, Texas: American Heart Association; 2005.

UK Cholesterol level targets available at: www.bhf.org.uk/youngpeople/uploaded/bhf_heartstats_2003_summary.pdf

Diabetes: the cost of diabetes: Fact sheet N°236. Revised September 2002. www.who.int

World Health Organisation cancer figures available at: www.who.int/cancer/en/

UK Cancer Statistics available at: http://info.cancerresearchuk.org/cancerstats/?a=5441

UK Office for National Statistics Mortality Statistics: Cause, 2004 available at: www.statistics.gov.uk/statbase/Product.asp?vlnk=618

US National Center for Chronic Disease Prevention and Health Promotion available at : www.cdc.gov/nccdphp/index.htm

Parkin DM, et al. Global Cancer Statistics, 2002. CA Cancer J Clin 2005;55;74-108.

World Health Organization obesity figures available at: www.who.int/dietphysicalactivity/publications/facts/obesity/en/

US overweight and obesity rates available at: www.cdc.gov/nchs/products/pubs/pubd/hestats/obese03_04/overwght_adult_03.htm

Canadian Consumer Trends in Obesity and Food Consumption February 2004

Prentice AM. The emerging epidemic of obesity in developing countries. International Journal of Epidemiology 2006 35(1):93-99; doi:10.1093/ije/dyi272

Canadian Institute for Health Information. (2004). Improving the health of Canadians – Summary report. Retrieved February 27, 2004 from www.cihi.ca.

European Obesity rates: www.euro.who.int/document/mediacentre/fs1305e.pdf World Health Organisation

EFFO and NOF (1997) Who are candidates for prevention and treatment for osteoporosis? Osteoporos Int 7:1. Available at: www.osteofound.org/press_centre/fact_sheet.html#general

Ray NF, et al. 3rd (1997) Medical expenditures for the treatment of osteoporotic fractures in the United States in 1995: report from the National Osteoporosis Foundation. J Bone Miner Res 12:24.

Mead PS, et al. Food-related illness and death in the United States. Emerg Infect Dis 1999;5:607-25.

Hall G, et al. Estimating foodborne gastroenteritis, Australia. Emerg Infect Dis 2005;11:1257-64.

Adak GK, et al. Trends in indigenous foodborne disease and deaths, England and Wales: 1992 to 2000. Gut 2002;51:832-41.

Bennett JW, et al. Mycotoxins. Clinical Microbiology Reviews, July 2003, p. 497–516 DOI: 10.1128/CMR.16.3.497–516.2003

Bennett JW et al. Mycotoxins. Clinical Microbiology Reviews, July 2003, p. 497–516 Vol. 16, No. 3. 0893-8512/03/$08.000 DOI: 10.1128/CMR.16.3.497–516.2003

US Food and Drug Administration. Foodborne Pathogenic Microorganisms and Natural Toxins Handbook: Clostridium botulinum. www.cfsan.fda.gov/~mow/chap2.html

Lindstrom M, et al. Hazard and control of group II (non-proteolytic) Clostridium botulinum in modern food processing. Int J Food Microbiol. 2006 Apr 15;108(1):92-104. Epub 2006 Feb 9.

The December 1995 issue of "FDA Consumer" has an article titled Botulism Toxin: a Poison That Can Heal which discusses Botulism toxin with an emphasis on its medical uses.

Drug-resistant Salmonella. Fact sheet N°139. Revised April 2005. www.who.int

Medus C,et al. Salmonella outbreaks in restaurants in Minnesota, 1995 through 2003: evaluation of the role of infected food workers. J Food Prot. 2006 Aug;69(8):1870-8.

Takkinen J, et al. A nationwide outbreak of multiresistant Salmonella Typhimurium in Finland due to contaminated lettuce from Spain, May 2005. Euro Surveill. 2005 Jun 30;10(6):E050630.1.

Colborn T. A Case for Revisiting the Safety of Pesticides: A Closer Look at Neurodevelopment. Environ Health Perspect. 2006 January; 114(1): 10–17. Published online 2005 September 7. doi: 10.1289/ehp.7940.

Dioxins and their effects on human health (World Health Organisation)
www.who.int/mediacentre/factsheets/fs225/en/

Hodges JR et al. The global diet: trade and novel infections. Globalization and Health
2005, 1:4 doi:10.1186/1744-8603-1-4. This article is available from:
www.globalizationandhealth.com/content/1/1/4

UK Additives E numbers listing available at:
www.food.gov.uk/safereating/chemsafe/additivesbranch/enumberlist

Lawrence G, et al. Acrylamide: review of toxicity data and dose-response analyses for
cancer and noncancer effects. Crit Rev Toxicol. 2006 Jul-Aug;36(6-7):481-608.

Vesper, H et al. Assessing human exposure to acrylamide. Environmental Exposure and
Health pp. 195-203.

Prof. Dr. Hanspeter Naegeli (Project Leader). HEATOX: Health risks from heat-treated
foods and food products. Weitere Informationen. Universität Zürich, 1. November 2005,
Impressum. Accessed at : www.research-projects.unizh.ch/p4862.htm

Gokmen, V. et al. Study of colour and acrylamide formation in coffee, wheat flour and
potato chips during heating. Food Chemistry, (2006) 99 (2) 238-243. DOI:
10.1016/j.foodchem.2005.06.054

The HEATOX project available at:
www.slv.se/templatesHeatox/Heatox_Page.aspx?id=8428

Agency Approves First Use of Viruses as a Food Additive. The Associated Press.
Accessed on: August 19, 2006, Saturday, Late Edition - Final, Section A, Page 11. Also
available at: www.nytimes.com/

Shannon Copeland, et al. Acute Inflammatory Response to Endotoxin in Mice and
Humans. Clin Diagn Lab Immunol. American Society for Microbiology 2005 January;
12(1): 60–67. doi: 10.1128/CDLI.12.1.60-67.2005.

Oshima H, et al. Hyperplastic gastric tumors induced by activated macrophages in COX-
2/mPGES-1 transgenic mice. EMBO J. 2004 Apr 7; 23(7): 1669-1678.

Jeffrey M. Smith. Seeds of Deception: Exposing Industry and Government Lies About
the Safety of the Genetically Engineered Foods You're Eating. Yes! Books; Iowa.
September 2003.

See Ho MW. Horizontal Gene Transfer. The Hidden Hazards of Genetic Engineering,
TWN Biotechnology Series, Third World Network, 2001 (available fom the ISIS online
store); also Ho MW. Horizontal gene transfer and genetic engineering, SCOPES website,
AAAS, 2000.

Ho MW. Briefing to the Rt. Hon. Michael Meacher, Minister for the Environment on the
Special Safety Concerns of Transgenic Agriculture and Related Issues. April 1999 ;
published in Seminario Internacional sobtre Direcito da Biodiversidade, Revista cej:
Centro de estudos Judiciarios do Conselho da Justica Federal, Brasil, pp.120-6, 1999.

Mae-Wan Ho. Predicted hazard of gene therapy a reality. Science, News of the Week, 4
October 2002;ISIS Report, October 2002

CDC.1996b. Outbreak of trichinellosis associated with eating cougar jerky-Idaho, 1995.
Atlanta, Ga. Morb. Mort. Wkly. Rept. 45(10): 205-206. U.S. Dept. of Health and Human
Services, Centers for Disease Control and Prevention, Atlanta, Ga.

CDC. 1998. Foodborne outbreak of cryptosporidiosis - Spokane, Washington, 1997.
Morb. Mort. Wkly. Rept. 47: 565-567. U.S. Dept. of Health and Human Services, Centers
for Disease Control and Prevention, Atlanta, Ga.

Machi, T.et al. 1997. Severe chest pain due to gastric anisakiasis. Intern. Med. 36(1): 28-
30.

de Lalla, F.et al. 1992. Outbreak of Entamoeba histolytica and Giardia lamblia infections in travellers returning from the tropics. Infection. 20(2): 78-82.

Muraoka, A.,et al. 1996. Acute gastric anisakiasis: 28 cases during the last 10 years. Dig. Dis. Sci. 41: 2362-2365.

Raisanen, S., et al. 1985. Epidemic ascariasis—Evidence of transmission by imported vegetables. Scand. J. Prim. Health Care. 3(3): 189-191.

Institute of Food Technologists. S-045 -- Parasites and the Food Supply . Discusses the sources and incidence of human infection by foodborne parasites and new technologies being developed for prevention, detection, and inactivation. April 2002.56[4]: 72-81.

Farm antibiotics pose risk to human health . James Meikle. Thursday August 19, 1999. The Guardian. www.guardian.co.uk/antibiotics/Story/0,,201997,00.html

Quintin A. et al. Antibiotics and resistance in farm animals. Nutrition & Food Science. Aug 1999 Vol. 99 Issue: 4 p178 – 184. DOI: 10.1108/00346659910270918. Article available at : www.emeraldinsight.com/10.1108/00346659910270918

Bonné, J. Livestock antibiotics found in waterways. 2004. Available at: www.msnbc.msn.com/id/6299642/

Carlson et al. Antibiotics used for growth in food animals making their way into waterways. 2004. Available at: www.newswise.com/p/articles/view/507755/

Environmental Media Services. Agricultural use of antibiotics. 2004. Available at: www.ems.org/antibiotics/antibiotics_food.html

O'Brien. Foodborne zoonoses. BMJ 2005;331;1217-1218. doi:10.1136/bmj.331.7527.1217. Downloaded from bmj.com on 21/02/2006

Food and Drug Administration Pesticide Program Residue Monitoring 2003. Data available from FDA's website, at www.cfsan.fda.gov.

Kimball et al. Trade related infections: farther, faster, quieter. Globalization and Health 2005, 1:3 doi:10.1186/1744-8603-1-3

Thomas D. Meat and dairy: where have the minerals gone? Food Magazine 72 10 Jan/Mar 2006

Nutraceutical new products accessed at: www.nutraceuticalsworld.com/articles/2006/09/new-products.php

IFT (2005) Functional Foods: Opportunities and Challenges. Chicago, IL, USA: Institute of Food Technologists.

Brower V. A nutraceutical a day may keep the doctor away. Science and SocietyEMBO Rep. 2005 August; 6(8): 708–711. doi: 10.1038/sj.embor.7400498.

Edmonds Institute. "Biohazards: The Next Generation?". November 2000. 20319-92nd Avenue West. Edmonds, Washington, 98020, e-mail: beb@igc.org

Cody V, et al. Plant Flavonoids in Biology and Medicine II: Biochemical, Cellular, and Medicinal Properties. Alan R Liss, Inc, NY, 1988.

Lampe JW. Health effects of vegetables and fruits: assessing mechanisms of action in human experimental studies. Am J Clin Nutr 1999;70(suppl)475S-90S.

Messina M, Messina V. Nutritional Implications of Dietary Phytochemicals. In: Dietary Phytochemicals in Cancer Prevention and Treatment. Plenum Press. New York, 1996.

Pariza M. Functional foods: technology, functionality, and health benefits. Nutrition Today. 1999;34:150–151.

Steinmetz KA, Potter JD. Vegetables, fruit, and cancer.II: Mechanisms Cancer Causes and Control 1991;2:427–442.

Van Poppel G, Goldbohm RA. Epidemiologic evidence for beta-carotene and cancer prevention. Am J Clin Nutr 1995;62:1393S-1402S.

Toyoshima, T et al. Functional Food in Japan--Status and Trend . Feb. 9, 2004. Available http://websrv2.tekes.fi/opencms/opencms/OhjelmaPortaali/Kaynnissa/ELITE/fi/Dokumenttiarkisto/Viestinta_ja_aktivointi/Julkaisut/Functional_Food_in_Japan_-Status_and_Trend.doc

Some Figures about Nanotechnology R&D in Europe and Beyond, European Commission, December 2005

Helmuth Kaiser Consultancy, Nanotechnology in Food and Food Processing Industry Worldwide, 2004. Report available at: www.hkc22.com/nanofood.html

Bread with fish oil information available at: www.foodscience.afisc.csiro.au/foodfacts/foodfacts11-fishoil.htm

The nanotechnology used to fight cholesterol available at: www.nutralease.com/technology.asp

Delivery of nutrients without changing food taste available at: www.biodeliverysciences.com/bioralnutrients.html

BASF & AQUANOVA functional foods available at: www.aquanova.de/partner.htm#degussa

How super-cows and nanotechnology will make ice cream healthy, Daily Telegraph Accessed: (21.8.05); available at: www.telegraph.co.uk/money/main.jhtml?xml=/money/2005/08/21/ccunil21.xml&menuId=242&sSheet=/money/2005/08/21/ixcoms.html

US Food and Drug Administration – Nanotechnology available at: www.fda.gov/nanotechnology/

Fergusson R. The Penguin Dictionary of Proverbs (Paperback). Penguin Books (1983)

Prophet Mohammed on food available at: www.islamic-world.net/papers/islamic.htm

Avicenna (Ibne Sina). Canon of Medicine (Al-Qanun fi'l at-Tibb). Abjad Book Designers & Builders (1999)

Arnold H Glasgow quotation available at: www.inspirationalquotes4u.com/glasgowquotes/index.html

Farshchi HR, et al. Decreased thermic effect of food after an irregular compared with a regular meal pattern in healthy lean women. Int J Obes Relat Metab Disord. 2004 May;28(5):653-60.

Farshchi HR, et al. Beneficial metabolic effects of regular meal frequency on dietary thermogenesis, insulin sensitivity, and fasting lipid profiles in healthy obese women. Am J Clin Nutr. 2005 Jan;81(1):16-24.

Farshchi HR, et al. Regular meal frequency creates more appropriate insulin sensitivity and lipid profiles compared with irregular meal frequency in healthy lean women. Eur J Clin Nutr. 2004 Jul;58(7):1071-7.

Zerva A, et al. Effect of Eating Frequency on Body Composition in 9 - 11-Year-Old Children. Int J Sports Med. 2006 Oct 6;

Howarth NC, et al. Eating patterns and dietary composition in relation to BMI in younger and older adults. Int J Obes (Lond). 2006 Sep 5;

Adelle Davis quote available at: www.quotationspage.com/quote/1677.html

Adelle Davis. Let's Get Well, Harcourt, Brace & World 1965, Chapter 1, page 5

Datamonitor. The Future of Mealtimes. Report Published: Jun-05 Product Code: DMCM2364. Available at: www.datamonitor.com

Los Angeles Times; The Breakfast Hype by Andreas von Bubnoff.. September 18, 2006. Accessed: 12:19 PM PDT, October 20, 2006 and available at: www.latimes.com/features/health/la-he-breakfast18sep18,0,2213526.story?page=1&coll=la-home-health

Third National Health and Nutrition Examination Survey (NHANES III). National Center for Health Statistics. Available at: www.cdc.gov/nchs/products/elec_prods/subject/nhanes3.htm

de Castro JM. The time of day of food intake influences overall intake in humans. J Nutr. 2004 Jan;134(1):104-11.

Farshchi HR, et al. Deleterious effects of omitting breakfast on insulin sensitivity and fasting lipid profiles in healthy lean women. Am J Clin Nutr. 2005 Feb;81(2):388-96.

InteliHealth: Does Nighttime Noshing Make You Fat? www.intelihealth.com/IH/ihtIH/WSI/9273/35323/432544.html?d=dmtHMSContent

National Institute of Diabetes and Digestive and Kidney Diseases (NIDDK) of the National Institutes of Health: Weight-loss and Nutrition Myths: http://win.niddk.nih.gov/publications/myths.htm

Yunsheng M, et al. Association between Eating Patterns and Obesity in a Free-living US Adult Population. Am J Epidemiol 2003; 158:85-92.

Ello-Martin JA, et al. The influence of food portion size and energy density on energy intake: implications for weight management. Am J Clin Nutr. 2005 Jul;82(1 Suppl):236S-241S.

Rolls BJ, et al. Reductions in portion size and energy density of foods are additive and lead to sustained decreases in energy intake. Am J Clin Nutr. 2006 Jan;83(1):11-7.

de Castro JM. Macronutrient and dietary energy density influences on the intake of free-living humans. Appetite. 2006 Jan;46(1):1-5. Epub 2005 Sep 19.

Wansink B, Kim J. Bad Popcorn in Big Buckets: Portion Size Can Influence Intake as Much as Taste. Journal of Nutrition Education and Behavior- 2005 09 (Vol. 37, Issue 5)

Otsuka R, et al. Eating fast leads to obesity: findings based on self-administered questionnaires among middle-aged Japanese men and women. J Epidemiol. 2006 May;16(3):117-24.

Katz, DL The Addictive Properties of Food! Yale-Griffin Prevention Research Center; Preventive Medicine Column. 1999

Colantuoni C,et al. Evidence That Intermittent, Excessive Sugar Intake Causes Endogenous Opioid Dependence. OBESITY RESEARCH Vol. 10 No. 6 p.478-88 June 2002.

Wang Gene-Jack, et al. Similarity Between Obesity and Drug Addiction as Assessed by Neurofunctional Imaging: A Concept Review. Journal of Addictive Diseases (The Haworth Medical Press, an imprint of The Haworth Press, Inc.) Vol. 23,No. 3, 2004, pp. 39-53.

Sorensen LB, et al.Effect of sensory perception of foods on appetite and food intake: a review of studies on humans. Int J Obes Relat Metab Disord. 2003 Oct;27(10):1152-66.

Smeets AJ, et al. Oral exposure and sensory-specific satiety. Physiol Behav. 2006 Sep 30;89(2):281-6. Epub 2006 Jul 27.

Household Food Security in the United States, 2004. By Mark Nord, Margaret Andrews, and Steven Carlson . Economic Research Report No. (ERR11) 65 pp, October 2005. Available online at: www.ers.usda.gov/Publications/err11/

World Development Indicators 2006. The World Bank. Available online at: www.worldbank.org/

State of Food Insecurity in the World 2005. Food and Agriculture Organization of the United Nations.PDF available at: www.fao.org/docrep/008/a0200e/a0200e00.htm

Aristotle ethics available at: www.constitution.org/ari/ethic_02.htm

Stitt PA. Fighting the Food Giants (Paperback). Natural Pr; Rev/Update edition (February 1983)

Stitt PA. Beating the Food Giants (Paperback). Natural Press (June 1982)

Science behind the Brands: Proctor & Gamble: Company news accessed 27/10/2006 http://pg.com/company/index.jhtml;jsessionid=YACKVEPKOFFZLQFIAJ4HK0GAVA BHO3MQ

Pringles product information available at: www.pringles.co.uk/information/lineup2.html#one

Pringles advertising. Proctor &Gamble: http://pg.com/product_card/prod_card_food_bev.jhtml

Lustig RH. Childhood obesity: behavioral aberration or biochemical drive? Reinterpreting the First Law of Thermodynamics. Nat Clin Pract Endocrinol Metab. 2006 Aug;2(8):447-58.

Yeomans MR, et al. Opioid peptides and the control of human ingestive behaviour. Neurosci Biobehav Rev. 2002 Oct;26(6):713-28.

Harrold JA, et al. The cannabinoid system: a role in both the homeostatic and hedonic control of eating? Br J Nutr. 2003 Oct;90(4):729-34.

Manier J, Callahan P, Alexander D. The Oreo, Obesity and Us. Chicago Tribune. Published August 2005

The Oreo Case. Ban Trans Fats. Available online at: www.bantransfats.com/theoreocase.html

Cookies in the US. Packaged facts. Market research report August 1, 2006 146 Pages Pub ID: LA1209582

Dietary Reference Intakes for Water, Potassium, Sodium, Chloride, and Sulfate. Food and Nutrition Board (FNB). The National Academic Press; Washington, D.C. 2004

PDR® Family Guide to Nutrition and Health. Thompson Healthcare 2004

Mintel International Group Ltd. Market Intelligence Food and Drink, Market Intelligence: UK Report: Dieting - UK - January 2006. Available at: http://reports.mintel.com/index.html

Mintel International Group Ltd. Market Intelligence Food and Drink, Market Intelligence: UK Report: Snacking on the Go - UK - April 2004. Available at: http://reports.mintel.com/index.html

Wansink B, et al. Bad popcorn in big buckets: portion size can influence intake as much as taste. J Nutr Educ Behav. 2005 Sep-Oct;37(5):242-5.

Hetherington MM, et al. Understanding variety: tasting different foods delays satiation. Physiol Behav. 2006 Feb 28;87(2):263-71. Epub 2006 Jan 6

Wansink B, et al. Ice cream illusions bowls, spoons, and self-served portion sizes. Am J Prev Med. 2006 Sep;31(3):240-3.

Wansink B, et al. Bottomless bowls: why visual cues of portion size may influence intake. Obes Res. 2005 Jan;13(1):2. Obes Res. 2005 Jan;13(1):93-100.

McArdale WD, Katch FI, Katch VL. Exercise Physiology: Energy, Nutrition, and Human Performance. 5th ed. Lippincott Williams & Wilkins, Philadelphia, 2001.

Rolls BJ, et al. Increasing the portion size of a packaged snack increases energy intake in men and women. Appetite. 2004 Feb;42(1):63-9.

FAO (Food and Agriculture Organisation of theUnited Nations). A Treaty on plant genetic resources. Agriculture 21 Magazine - Spotlight 2001. Published December 2001. Available at: www.fao.org/ag/magazine/0112sp3.htm

Kellogg's product information www.kellogs.com & available breakfast cereal range accessed 28/10/2006 at: www.kelloggs.com/cgi-bin/brandpages/product.pl?company=3&brand=162&template=cereal

Schwartz B. The Paradox of Choice: Why More Is Less. HarperCollins; New York. 2005

Kraak V, et al. How marketers reach young consumers: Implications for nutrition education and health promotion campaigns. Family Economics and Nutrition Review 1998, 11:31-41

Fischer PM, et al. Brand logo recognition by children aged 3 to 6 years. Mickey Mouse and Old Joe the Camel. JAMA 1991, 266:3145-3148.

Perry CL. The relationship between "share of voice" and "share of market" and implications for youth health promotion. Health Education 1998, 29:206-212.

Kotz K,et al. Food advertisements during children's Saturday morning television programming: Are they consistent with dietary recommendations? J Am Diet Assoc 1994, 94:1296-1300.

Coon KA, et al. Television and children's consumption patterns. A review of the literature. Minerva Pediatr 2002, 54:423-436.

Mary Story et al. Food Advertising and Marketing Directed at Children and Adolescents in the US. International Journal of Behavioral Nutrition and Physical Activity 2004, 1:3. This article is available from: www.ijbnpa.org/content/1/1/3

Food Commission UK Press release: Monday 5th April 2004: Food Commission welcomes BBC promise to cease Tweenies abuse. Available at: www.foodcomm.org.uk/press_BBC_04.htm

Hawkes C. Marketing Food to Children: The Global Regulatory Environment. Geneva: World Health Organization. 2004.

M&M's film tie-in available at: www.confectionerynews.com/news/ng.asp?id=67445-mars-m-m-s-chocolate

McGinnis MJ, et al. Food Marketing to Children and Youth Threat or Opportunity? Committee on Food Marketing and the Diets of Children and Youth. Food and Nutrition Board. Institute of Medicine of the National Acadamies. The National Academic Press. Washington, D.C. 2006. www.nap.edu

Rothman, RL, et al, "Patient Understanding of Food Labels: The Role of Literacy and Numeracy," American Journal of Preventive Medicine 2006; 31 (5): doi: 10.1016/j.amepre.2006.07.025

Wansink, B. How Do Front and Back Package Labels Influence Beliefs About Health Claims?.Journal of Consumer Affairs 37 (2), 305-316.doi: 10.1111/j.1745-6606.2003.tb00455.x. 2003

National Consumer Council. Healthy competition: how supermarkets can affect your chances of a healthy diet. Report available at : www.ncc.org.uk/food/index.htm

Campaigners against the Tesco supermarket global company. Details available at: www.tescopoly.org

Tesco International facts and figures; available at:
www.tescocorporate.com/factsheets.htm

Nestle M. New York University, Nutrition, Food Studies, and Public Health.
www.foodpolitics.com/

Nestle M. Food company sponsorship of nutrition research and professional activities: a
conflict of interest? Public Health Nutrition: 4(5), 1015±1022. DOI:
10.1079/PHN2001253

Resources

www.britannica.com	Encyclopædia Britannica Online
www.glycemicindex.com/	Glycemic Index & Load resources
www.mendosa.com/gilists.htm	Glycemic Index & Load resources
www.foodcomm.org.uk/About_us.htm	The Food Commission
www.cdc.gov/	US Centres for Disease Control and Prevention
www.fda.gov/fdac/features/2003/503_fats.html	Trans fat content of foods
www.ars.usda.gov/main/main.htm	U.S. Department of Agriculture. Agricultural Research Service
www.nal.usda.gov/fnic/cgi-bin/nut_search.pl	USDA Nutrient Database
www.heartstats.org	British Heart Foundation Statistics Database
www.diabetes.org.uk/	Diabetes UK
www.foodstandards.gov.uk/	UK Food Standards Agency
www.food.gov.uk/safereating/chemsafe/additivesbranch/enumberlist	UK additives

Part four – R & R

Ovid – Metamorphoses. Translated by A. D. Melville. Book XI. Oxford University Press.
1998.

The Bible. King James Version, Ecclesiastes (Ch. V, v. 12)

Al-Hilali MT & Kahn MM. The Noble Qur'an; Translations of the Qur'an, Surat An-
Naba' (The News); Chapter 78 p.693, line 9. Darussalam, Riyad, Saudi Arabia, 1996.

Schwartz JR, et al. Shift work sleep disorder : burden of illness and approaches to
management. Drugs. 2006;66(18):2357-70

Phipps-Nelson J, et al. Daytime exposure to bright light, as compared to dim light,
decreases sleepiness and improves psychomotor vigilance performance. Sleep. 2003
Sep;26(6):695-700

Costa G, et al. Influence of flexibility and variability of working hours on health and
well-being. Chronobiol Int. 2006;23(6):1125-37

Yuriko DOI. An Epidemiologic Review on Occupational Sleep Research among
Japanese Workers. Industrial Health 43:1,3. 2005

Markov D, et al. Normal sleep and circadian rhythms: neurobiologic mechanisms
underlying sleep and wakefulness. Psychiatr Clin North Am. 2006 Dec;29(4):841-53;

Czeisler CA, et al. Circadian and sleep-dependent regulation of hormone release in
humans. Recent Prog. Horm. Res. 1999;54:97-130; discussion 130-2

Richardson G, et al. Hormonal and pharmacological manipulation of the circadian clock:
recent developments and future strategies. Sleep. 2000 May 1;23 Suppl 3:S77-85

Atkinson G, et al. Relationships between sleep, physical activity and human health. Physiol Behav. 2006 Oct 24;

Reid KJ, et al. Sleep: a marker of physical and mental health in the elderly. Am J Geriatr Psychiatry. 2006 Oct;14(10):860-6

Owens J, et al. Television-viewing habits and sleep disturbance in school children. Pediatrics. 1999 Sep;104(3):e27

Costa e Silva JA. Sleep disorders in psychiatry. Metabolism. 2006 Oct;55(10 Suppl 2):S40-4.

Gibson ES, et al. "Sleepiness" is serious in adolescence: two surveys of 3235 Canadian students. BMC Public Health. 2006 May 2;6:116

Thompson DA, et al. The association between television viewing and irregular sleep schedules among children less than 3 years of age. Pediatrics. 2005 Oct;116(4):851-6

Prinz P. Sleep, appetite, and obesity—What is the link? PLoS Med (2004) 1(3): e61.

Kripke DF, et al. Mortality associated with sleep duration and insomnia. Arch Gen Psychiatry. 2002;59:131–136

Heslop P, et al. Sleep duration and mortality: The effect of short or long sleep duration on cardiovascular and all-cause mortality in working men and women. Sleep Med. 2002;3:305–314

Taheri S, et al. Short sleep duration is associated with reduced leptin, elevated ghrelin, and increased body mass index—A population-based study. PLoS Med. 2004;3:e62

Chen MY, et al. Adequate sleep among adolescents is positively associated with health status and health-related behaviours. BMC Public Health. 2006 Mar 8;6:59

Ireland JL, et al. The relationship between sleeping problems and aggression, anger, and impulsivity in a population of juvenile and young offenders. J Adolesc Health. 2006 Jun;38(6):649-55

Mallon L, et al. High incidence of diabetes in men with sleep complaints or short sleep duration: a 12-year follow-up study of a middle-aged population. Diabetes Care. 2005 Nov;28(11):2762-7

Mallis MM, et al. Circadian rhythms, sleep, and performance in space. Aviat Space Environ Med. 2005 Jun;76(6 Suppl):B94-107

Doi Y. An epidemiologic review on occupational sleep research among Japanese workers. Ind Health. 2005 Jan;43(1):3-10

Hilliard RE. Music Therapy in Hospice and Palliative Care: a Review of the Empirical Data. eCAM 2005;2(2)173–178. doi:10.1093/ecam/neh076. Oxford University Press.

Resources

Travell JG & Simons OG. Myofascial Pain and Dysfunction: The Trigger Point Manual; Vol. II 2nd ed. Baltimore. Lippincott Williams and Wilkins 1992

Simons OG & Travell JG. Myofascial Pain and Dysfunction: The Trigger Point Manual; Vol. I 2nd ed. Baltimore. Lippincott Williams and Wilkins 1999

Part five – Made for motion

Cordain L, et al. Physical Activity, Energy Expenditure and Fitness: An Evolutionary Perpctive, Int. J. Sports Med., Vol. 19, pp.328-335; 1998

Cavagna GA, et al. Mechanical work in terrestrial locomotion: two basic mechanisms for minimising energy expenditure. Am J Physiol 1977; 233 R243-R61

Rodman PS, et al. Bioenergetics and the origin of hominoid bipedalism. Am J Phys Anthropol 1980; 52: 103-6

Lowes Dickinson G. The Greek View Of Life. 6th Ed. New York. 1909

Bouchard C, et al. Physical Activity, Fitness and Health: International Proceedings and Consensus Statement. Champaign. Il. Human Kinetics. 1994

Fernandez-Real JM & Ricart W. Insulin resistance and inflammation in an evolutionary perspective: the contribution of cytokine genotype/phenotype to thriftiness. Diabetologia 42: 1367–1374, 1999

Eaton SB, et al. Stone agers in the fast lane: chronic degenerative diseases in evolutionary perspective. Am J Med 84: 739–749, 1988

Kimm SY, et al. Decline in physical activity in black girls and white girls during adolescence. N Engl J Med. 2002; 347: 709–715

Bull F. Defining physical inactivity. Lancet. 2003; 361: 258–259

Yancey AK, et al. Physical inactivity and overweight among Los Angeles County adults. Am J Prev Med. 2004; 27: 146–152

Hakim AA,et al. Effects of walking on mortality among nonsmoking retired men. N Engl J Med. 1998; 338: 94–99

Manson JE, et al. Walking compared with vigorous exercise for the prevention of cardiovascular events in women. N Engl J Med. 2002; 347: 716–725

Lees SJ, et al. Sedentary death syndrome. Can J Appl Physiol. 2004; 29: 447–460

Hambrecht R,et al. Effect of exercise on coronary endothelial function in patients with coronary artery disease. N Engl J Med. 2000; 342: 454–460

Belardinelli R, et al. Exercise training intervention after coronary angioplasty: the ETICA trial. J Am Coll Cardiol. 2001; 37: 1891–1900

Schuler G, et al. Regular physical exercise and low-fat diet. Effects on progression of coronary artery disease. Circulation. 1992; 86: 1–11

Rauramaa R,et al. Effects of aerobic physical exercise on inflammation and atherosclerosis in men: the DNASCO study: a six-year randomized, controlled trial. Ann Intern Med. 2004; 140: 1007–1014

Darren E.R. Warburton, et al. Health benefits of physical activity: the evidence. CMAJ 2006;174(6):801-9

Nordstrom CK, et al. Leisure time physical activity and early atherosclerosis: the Los Angeles Atherosclerosis Study. Am J Med. 2003; 115: 19–25

Stewart KJ. Exercise training and the cardiovascular consequences of type 2 diabetes and hypertension: plausible mechanisms for improving cardiovascular health. J Am Med Assoc. 2002; 288: 1622–1631

Wannamethee SG, et al. Physical activity and hemostatic and inflammatory variables in elderly men. Circulation. 2002; 105: 1785–1790

Youth Risk Behavior Surveillance System, Youth Risk Behavior Surveillance-United States, 2003 MMWR 53(SS-2):1-29, 2004. Accessed 17 August 2005; www.cdc.gov/healthyyouth/yrbs/

Physical inactivity among children today at epidemic levels; Child Health News. Accessed 15 June 2007; Published: Thursday, 31-May-2007 www.news-medical.net/?id=25731

Prentice A, Jebb S (2006) TV and inactivity are separate contributors to metabolic risk factors in children. PLoS Med 3(12): e481. doi:10.1371/journal. pmed.0030481

World Health Organisation Physical Inactivity Statistics; accessed June 15 2007.
www.who.int/dietphysicalactivity/publications/facts/pa/en/

Leaf A. Every Day Is a Gift When You Are Over 100. National Geographic.

Davies D. The Centenarians of the Andes. 1st ed. Barrie and Jenkins Limited, London; 1975

Kannus P, et al. The effects of training, immobilisation and remobilisation on musculoskeletal tissue. 1. Training and immobilisation. Scandinavian Journal of Medicine and Science in Sports 2: 100-118. 1992

Kannus P, et al. The effects of training, immobilisation and remobilisation on musculoskeletal tissue. 2. Remobilisation and prevention of immobilisation hypotrophy. Scandinavian Journal of Medicine and Science in Sports 2: 164-176. 1992

Woo SL, et al. Mechanical peoperties of tendons and ligaments. II. Biorheology 19:397-408. 1982

Jackson A, Morrow J, Hill D, Dishman R. Physical activity for health and fitness. Champaign, IL; Human Kinetics. 282. 1999

Bergouignan A, et al. (2006) Effect of physical inactivity on the oxidation of saturated and monounsaturated dietary fatty acids: Results of a randomized trial. PLoS Clin Trials 1(5): e27. DOI: 10.1371/journal.pctr.0010027

Benefits of Physical Activity by World Health Organisation; Accessed 15/7/2007
www.who.int/moveforhealth/advocacy/information_sheets/benefits/en/index.html

Sapolsky RM. Why sebras don't get ulcers – A guide to stress, stress-related diseases, and coping. New York: Freeman. 2003

Cohen, N, ed. The Everything You Want to Know About Sports Encyclopedia: A Sports Illustrated for Kids Book. New York: Bantam Books, 1994

Kybartas, R. Fitness Is Religion: Keep the Faith. New York: Simon and Schuster, 1997

Berryman JW. The tradition of the "six things non-natural": exercise and medicine from Hippocrates through Ante-Bellum America. Med Sci Sports Exerc 1989;17:515-59.

Murray CL, et al. The global burden of disease. A comprehensive assessment of mortality and disability from diseases, injuries, and risk factors in 1990 and projected for 2020. World Health Organisation, World Bank, Harvard University. 1996

Allender S, et al. The Burden of physical activity-related ill health in the UK. J Epidemiol Community Health. 2007 Apr;61(4):344-8.

Dishman RK, et al. Treadmill exercise training augments brain norepinephrine response to familiar and novel stress. Brain Research Bulletin 42:399-406. 2000

O'Neal H, et al. Physical activity and depression: A quantitive synthesis. Unpublished manuscript, The University of Georgia. 2002

Yoo HS, et al. Antidepressant-like effects of physical activity vs. imipramine: Neonatal clomipramine model. Psychobiology 28: 540-549. 2000

Fox KR. Self Esteem, self-perceptions and exercise. International Journal of Sports Psychology 31 (2): 228-240. 2000

Martinsen EW, et al. Comparing aerobic with nonaerobic forms of exercise in the treatment of clinical depression: A randomised trial. Comprehensive Psychiatry 30 (July-August): 324-331. 1989

Steven N Blair, et al. The evolution of physical activity recommendations: how much is enough? Am J Clin Nutr 2004;79(suppl):913S–20S.

Ballor D, et al. Resting Metabolic Rate and coronary heart risk in aerobically and resistance trained women. Amercian Journal of Clinical Nutrition 1992; 56:968-74

Broeder C, et al. The effects of either high intensity resistance or endurance training on resting metabolic rate. American Journal of Clinical Nutrition 1992; 55:802-810

Campbell W, et al. Increased energy requirements and changes in body composition with resistance training in older adults. American Journal of Clinical Nutrition 1994; 60:167-75

Caspersen CJ, et al. Physical activity, exercise, and physical fitness: Definitions and distinctions for health-related research. Public Health Rep 1985;100:126-131

Jakicic JM, et al. Effect of exercise duration and intensity on weight loss in overweight, sedentary women: a randomized trial. JAMA 2003; 290:1323-30

Institute of Medicine. Dietary reference intakes for energy, carbohydrate, fiber, fat, fatty acids, cholesterol, protein, and amino acids. Washington, DC: National Academies Press, 2002

Wing RR, et al. Successful weight loss maintenance. Annu Rev Nutr 2001; 21:323-41

Resources

www.cdc.gov   Centers for Disease Control and Prevention

Part six – A silent revolution

Dahl R. Heavy Traffic Ahead: Car Culture Accelerates. Environ Health Perspect. 2005 April; 113(4): A238–A245

Dahl R. Population Equation – Balancing what we have with what we need. Environmental Health Perspectives. 2005 September; 113(9): A599-A605

Pattison N, Warren L. 2002 drug industry profits: hefty pharmaceutical company margins dwarf other industries. Washington (DC): Public Citizen Congress Watch; June 2003. Available: www.citizen.org/documents/Pharma_Report.pdf

Fortune 500: How the industries stack up. Fortune 2004;149(7):F26.

Centers for Medicare & Medicaid Services, National Health Accounts, at www.cms.hhs.gov/statistics/nhe/default.asp.

Mayer M (2005) When clinical trials are compromised: A perspective from a patient advocate. PLoS Med 2(11): e358.

Relman A. Separating continuing medical education from pharmaceutical marketing. JAMA 2001;285:2009-12.

Nestle M. New York University, Nutrition, Food Studies, and Public Health. www.foodpolitics.com/

OTC Pharmaceuticals. Market Report; 12th ed. Keynote Ltd December 2005

Appendices

Appendix I
Glossary of principal pollutants produced by industrial, domestic and traffic sources:

Sulphur Dioxide
Sulphur dioxide is an acidic gas, which is damaging to the environment and in ambient air cause harmful health effects.

Principal source:
Power stations (Domestic and industrial power generation)
The last 40 years have seen a decline in coal burning developed countries (though still a major problem in developing countries). As a result, ambient concentrations of this pollutant, for example in the United Kingdom, have decreased steadily over this period.

Health Effects:
Tiniest amounts reduce lung function and induce erratic coughing in those suffering from asthma and lung diseases.

Particle Matter (PM_{10})
Airborne particulate matter varies in size and is usually identified by the fraction of particulates in air by its size, is of major current concern. They are small enough to penetrate deep into the lungs and so potentially pose significant health risks. Larger particles meanwhile, are not readily inhaled, and are removed relatively efficiently from the air by sedimentation.

Principal course:
Road traffic emissions, particularly from diesel vehicles

Health Effects
Lung inflammation and a worsening of the condition of people with heart and lung diseases; Carry carcinogenic compounds into the lungs; Negatively affects blood viscosity; Decrease heart rate variability; Coronary heart disease risk increase

Carbon Monoxide
Carbon monoxide (CO) is a toxic gas. It survives in the atmosphere for a period of approximately one month before it is oxidised to carbon dioxide (CO_2).

Principal course:
Combustion process
Urban areas 90% from road traffic emissions
Hydrocarbon and organic oxidation

Health Effects
Prevents the transportation of oxygen by the blood and leads to reductions in supplies to major organs, like the heart and the brain

Nitrogen Dioxide (NO_2)
Nitrogen oxides are formed during high temperature combustion processes from the oxidation of nitrogen in the air or fuel.

Principal sources:
Road traffic emissions
In Europe 50% from traffic emissions
Power stations, heating plants and industrial processes
Health Effects :
Irritation of the lungs; reduced resistance to respiratory infections such
as influenza; increased incidence of acute respiratory illness in children

Ozone (O_3)

Ground level ozone (O_3), is a secondary pollutant produced by reaction between
nitrogen dioxide, hydrocarbons, and sunlight. Ozone levels are higher in rural
areas. Higher levels of ozone are generally observed during hot, still sunny,
summertime weather.

Health Effects
Irritation of the lung airways; Increased the symptoms of those
suffering from asthma and lung diseases; Increased risk of blood
pressure; Higher risks of cardiovascular diseases

Volatile Organic Compounds (VOCs)

VOCs are released in vehicle exhaust gases either as unburned fuels or as
combustion products, and are emitted by the evaporation of solvents and motor
fuels.

Benzene is a constituent of petrol and is released by the distribution and
combustion of it, and accounts for 70% of European emissions in the
atmosphere.

1,3-butadiene is also emitted from fuel combustion of petrol but also
diesel vehicles. 1, 3-butadiene is an important chemical in certain industrial
processes, particularly the manufacture of synthetic rubber.

Health Effects:
Cancer; Central nervous system disorders; Liver and kidney damage;
Reproductive disorders; Birth defects

Toxic Organic Micro pollutants (TOMPs)

They are produced by the incomplete combustion of fuels and are complex
arrangements of chemicals. They have wide-ranging detrimental effects on
health and even in smallest amounts, are highly toxic or carcinogenic. They
include PolyAromatic Hydrocarbons (PAHs); Polychlorinated Biphenyls
(PCBs); Dioxins; Furans

Health Effects
Wide ranging and include: Cancer risks; Reduced immune system;
Nervous system disorders; Interference with child development

Lead and Heavy Metals

Particulate lead in air is produced by fossil fuel combustion (including vehicles),
metal processing industries, waste incineration, and the manufacture of batteries
(largest source). The smallest amounts are harmful to health.

Health Effects

Adverse effects in infants, young children, unborn babies through their mothers; Neurological damage in children; Respiratory diseases; Impaired mental function; Visual-motor performance; Memory problems; Decreased attention span

Acid Deposition

Sulphur dioxide and nitrogen oxides can also react with the moisture in air to form acids. They can travel long distances and eventually be deposited in the environment as what is commonly call acid rain. Acid rain can have harmful impacts on the environment.

It affects freshwater lakes and the wildlife that depend upon them. It also affects trees by harming leaves and soil, and it damages buildings made of limestone and marble.

Appendix II
Plant origin sources of the 9 Essential Amino Acids

Histidine: Apple, pomegranates, alfalfa, beetroots, carrots, celery, cucumber, endive, garlic, radish, spinach, turnip greens.

Valine: Apples, almonds, pomegranates, beetroots, carrots, celery, lettuce, okra, parsley, parsnips, squash, tomatoes, turnips, nutritional yeast.

Tryptophan: Alfalfa, Brussels sprouts, carrots, celery, chives, endive, fennel, beans, spinach, turnips, nutritional yeast.

Threnoine: Papayas, alfalfa sprouts, carrots, green leafy vegetables such as celery, collards, kale, and lettuce, beans, and sea vegetables.

Phenylalanine: Apples, pineapples, beetroots, carrots, parsley, spinach, tomatoes, nutritional yeast.

Methionine: Apples, pineapples, Brazil nuts, Brussels sprouts, cabbage, cauliflower, chives, garlic, horseradish, kale, watercress.

Lysine: Apples, apricots, grapes, papayas, pears, alfalfa, beets, carrots, celery, cucumber, parsley, spinach, turnip greens.

Leucine: Avocados, papayas, olives, coconut, sunflower seeds.

Isoleucine: Avocados, papayas, olives, coconut, sunflower seeds.

Appendix III
Vitamins and Minerals

Vitamin	Best sources	Health benefits
	Fat soluble vitamins	
Vitamin A & **Beta carotene**	Milk, eggs, cheese, butter, chicken, liver Plant sources: Orange, deep yellow, dark green leafy vegetables, and fruit;	Antioxidant; protects cells from damage by biochemical reactions; essential for growth and development; maintains healthy vision, skin, and

	the body converts beta carotene in these sources into vitamin A	reproductive functions
Vitamin D	Liver, butter, fatty fish, egg yolks Sunlight	Essential for formation of bones and teeth; increases calcium absorption
Vitamin E	Vegetable oils, whole grains, wheat germ, nuts, seeds, leafy green vegetables	Antioxidant; protects cells from damage by biochemical reactions. helps create blood cells, muscles, and lung and nerve tissue; boosts the immune system
Vitamin K	Dark-green leafy vegetables, fruits; also found in cereals, dairy products, and meat	Important in blood clotting
	Water soluble vitamins	
Vitamin C	Citrus fruits, tomatoes, broccoli, green peppers, strawberries, melons, cabbage, and leafy green vegetables; vitamin C is destroyed when foods are overcooked or cooked in large amounts of water	Antioxidant; necessary for healthy bones, teeth, and skin; helps in wound healing ; important in collagen synthesis
Vitamin B$_1$ (thiamine)	Whole grains, nuts, legumes, fruits, vegetables, enriched breads and cereals, pork, and liver	Helps convert food into energy; removal of carbon dioxide
Vitamin B$_2$ (riboflavin)	Meats, fish, whole grains, wheat germ, dark green vegetables, milk products, enriched breads, cereals, pasta	Helps in energy production and other chemical processes in the body; helps maintain healthy eyes, skin, and nerve function
Vitamin B$_3$ (niacin)	Whole grains, legumes, peanuts, milk products, meat, poultry, fish, nuts, broccoli, green peas, green beans	Helps convert food into energy; helps maintain proper brain function; aids in manufacture of fatty acids
Vitamin B$_6$ (pyridoxine)	Whole wheat products, meat, fish, nuts, cereal, seeds, green beans,	Helps produce essential amino acids; helps convert protein into energy

	bananas, green leafy vegetables, potatoes	
Vitamin B$_{12}$ (cobalamin)	Meats, dairy products, eggs, liver, nutritional yeast, fortified cereal, soy milk	Helps DNA synthesis (production of the genetic material of cells); helps convert carbohydrates and fatty acids into energy; helps with formation of red blood cells and maintenance of central nervous system; helps make amino acids building blocks of proteins)
Folic acid (folate)	Dark green leafy vegetables, fruits, dried beans and peas, eggs, milk products, liver	Helps DNA synthesis (production of the genetic material of cells); essential in first 3 months of pregnancy for preventing birth defects; helps in red blood cell formation; protects against heart disease
Pantothenic Acid	Legumes, whole grains, meat, fish, poultry	Aids in energy production; aids in the manufacture of fatty acids; participates in a wide variety of other biochemical processes
Biotin	Legumes, vegetables, nuts, meats, liver, egg yolk	Required for fat synthesis and amino acids metabolism; Energy production

Mineral	**Best sources**	**Health benefits**
	Minerals – (major)	
Calcium	Dark green leafy vegetables, dried legumes, dairy products, sardines (with bones), salmon	The most abundant mineral in the body, 99 percent is in bones; essential for building bones and teeth and maintaining bone strength; important in muscle function
Phosphorus	Grain products, meat, dairy products, poultry, fish	Essential for building strong bones and teeth; helps in formation of genetic material; helps in energy production and storage; loss of calcium
Potassium	Leafy green vegetables, fruits, beans, nuts, grains, seeds, meats, milk	Essential for maintaining balance of body fluids, transmitting nerve signals, and producing energy
Sodium	Table salt, vegetables,	Essential for maintaining normal

	animal foods, some bottled waters	blood pressure and balance of body fluids and for transmitting nerve signals, and relax muscles
Chloride	Table salt, some vegetables and fruit, eggs, meat, milk	Is a component of stomach acid; aids in maintaining body fluid balance in cells
Magnesium	Leafy green vegetables, nuts, whole grains, dried peas and beans, dairy products, fish, meat, poultry	Essential for healthy nerve and muscle function and bone formation; may help prevent premenstrual syndrome (PMS), general metabolic processes
Minerals – (minor)		
Copper	Whole grains, nuts, liver, oysters, drinking water	Essential for making haemoglobin (oxygen carrying protein in red blood cells) and collagen (a protein in connective tissue); essential for healthy heart functioning; helps in energy production; helps in absorption of iron from digestive tract
Iron	Meat, poultry, fish, dried beans, nuts, dried fruits, leafy green vegetables, whole-grain and enriched grain products	Helps in energy production; helps to carry oxygen in the bloodstream and to transfer oxygen to muscles
Selenium	Fish, meat, whole-grain breads and cereals	Antioxidant; essential for healthy functioning of the heart muscle; protects cells against harmful reactions involving oxygen; aids in detoxifying toxic substances functions closely with vitamin E
Zinc	Meats, poultry, oysters, eggs, legumes, nuts, milk, yogurt, whole-grain cereals	Is necessary for cell reproduction and tissue repair and growth; production of sperm and the male hormone testosterone
Chromium	Whole grains, brewer's yeast, nuts, dried beans	Works with insulin to promote carbohydrate and fat breakdown and use

Appendix IV
Additives

Commonly found additives in your food, to avoid:

Additives	What to look for on the label
Preservatives & synthetic antioxidants	Ascorbic acid, citric acid, sodium benzoate, calcium propionate, sodium erythorbate, sodium nitrite, calcium sorbate, potassium sorbate, tocopherols, BHA, BHT, EDTA.
Sweeteners	Sugar, sucrose, glucose, fructose, sorbitol, mannitol, corn syrup, high fructose corn syrup, saccharin, aspartame, sucralose, acesulfame potassium (acesulfame-K), neotame
Colour	FD&C Blue Nos. 1 and 2, FD&C Green No. 3, FD&C Red Nos. 3 and 40, FD&C Yellow Nos. 5 and 6, Orange B, Citrus Red No. 2, annatto extract, beta-carotene, grape skin extract, cochineal extract or carmine, paprika oleoresin, caramel colour, fruit and vegetable juices, saffron
Flavourings and flavour enhancers	Natural flavouring, artificial flavour, and spices, monosodium glutamate (MSG), hydrolyzed soy protein, autolyzed yeast extract, disodium guanylate or inosinate
Fat substitutes	Olestra, cellulose gel, carrageenan, polydextrose, modified food starch, micro articulated egg white protein, guar gum, xanthan gum, whey protein concentrate
Nutrients	Thiamine hydrochloride, riboflavin (Vitamin B2), niacin, niacin amide, folate or folic acid, beta carotene, potassium iodide, iron or ferrous sulphate, alpha tocopherols, ascorbic acid, Vitamin D, amino acids (L-tryptophan, L-lysine, L-leucine, L-methionine)
Emulsifiers and emulsifying salts	Soy lecithin, mono- and diglycerides, egg yolks, polysorbates, sorbitan monostearate
Stabilisers and thickeners	Gelatine, pectin, guar gum, carrageenan, xanthan gum, whey

Acidity regulator	Lactic acid, citric acid, ammonium hydroxide, sodium carbonate
Leavening Agents	Baking soda, monocalcium phosphate, calcium carbonate
Anti-caking agents	Calcium silicate, iron ammonium citrate, silicon dioxide
Humectants	Glycerine, sorbitol
Raising agent	Calcium sulphate, ammonium phosphate
Flour treatment agents	Ammonium sulphate, azodicarbonamide, L-cysteine
Firming Agents	Calcium chloride, calcium lactate
Enzyme Preparations	Enzymes, lactase, papain, rennet, chymosin
Gases	Carbon dioxide, nitrous oxide

UK Additives E numbers listing available at:
www.food.gov.uk/safereating/chemsafe/additivesbranch/enumberlist